Health Inequalities and People w

Health Inequalities and People with Intellectual Disabilities

Eric Emerson

Professor of Disability Population Health, Centre for Disability Research and Policy, University of Sydney, Australia

Professor of Disability and Health Research, Centre for Disability Research, Lancaster University, UK

Chris Hatton

Professor of Psychology, Health and Social Care, Centre for Disability Research, Lancaster University, UK

Co-Director of Improving Health and Lives, Public Health England

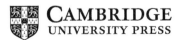

YORK ST. JOHN
LIBRARY & INFORMATION
SERVICES

CAMBRIDGE
UNIVERSITY PRESS

CAMBRIDGE
UNIVERSITY PRESS

University Printing House, Cambridge CB2 8BS, United Kingdom

Published in the United States of America by Cambridge University Press, New York

Cambridge University Press is part of the University of Cambridge.

It furthers the University's mission by disseminating knowledge in the pursuit of education, learning and research at the highest international levels of excellence.

www.cambridge.org
Information on this title: www.cambridge.org/9780521133142

© Eric Emerson and Chris Hatton

First published 2014

Printed in the United Kingdom by CPI Group Ltd, Croydon CR0 4YY

A catalogue record for this publication is available from the British Library

Library of Congress Cataloguing in Publication data
Emerson, Eric, 1953– author.
Health inequalities and people with intellectual disabilities / Eric Emerson, Chris Hatton.
    p. ; cm.
Includes bibliographical references and index.
ISBN 978-0-521-13314-2 (pbk.)
I. Hatton, Chris (Professor), author.   II. Title.
[DNLM: 1. Health Status Disparities.   2. Intellectual Disability.   3. Disabled Persons–psychology.   4. Socioeconomic Factors. WA 300]
RC570
362.3–dc23
2013023445

ISBN 978-0-521-13314-2 Paperback

Every effort has been made in preparing this book to provide accurate and up-to-date information which is in accord with accepted standards and practice at the time of publication. Although case histories are drawn from actual cases, every effort has been made to disguise the identities of the individuals involved. Nevertheless, the authors, editors and publishers can make no warranties that the information contained herein is totally free from error, not least because clinical standards are constantly changing through research and regulation. The authors, editors and publishers therefore disclaim all liability for direct or consequential damages resulting from the use of material contained in this book. Readers are strongly advised to pay careful attention to information provided by the manufacturer of any drugs or equipment that they plan to use.

Contents

List of abbreviations   *page* vii

1   People with intellectual disabilities   1
     Understanding intellectual disability   1
     Mapping models of intellectual disability on to health and
         health inequalities   3
     The capabilities framework   4
     Classifying intellectual disabilities   18
     The epidemiology of intellectual disabilities   19
     Summary   24

2   Health and health inequalities   25
     Health: conceptualisation and measurement   25
     Health inequalities   35
     The determinants of health and health inequalities   36

3   The health of people with intellectual disabilities   40
     Evaluating the evidence base   40
     General indicators of health   49
     Specific health conditions and impairments   53
     Summary and conclusions   64

4   Applying a health inequalities perspective   66
     Health inequalities   66
     Determinants of the health inequalities experienced by
         people with intellectual disabilities   67
     Conclusions   81

5   Addressing the health inequalities faced by people with
     intellectual disabilities   83
     Public health perspectives on improving health and
         reducing health inequalities   83
     Level 1: counselling and education   87
     Level 2: clinical interventions   94
     Level 3: long-lasting protective interventions   96

*Level 4: changing the context to make individuals' default
decisions healthy*   100
Level 5: socio-economic factors   103
Conclusions   105

6   Conclusions   108
Challenges ahead   110
A final word   115

References   117
Index   161

Abbreviations

AAIDD	American Association on Intellectual and Developmental Disabilities
ICD	International Statistical Classification of Diseases and Related Health Problems (WHO)
ICF	International Classification of Functioning, Disability and Health (WHO)
SEP	socio-economic position
UNCRPD	UN Convention on the Rights of Persons with Disabilities

People with intellectual disabilities

This opening chapter is designed to sketch some of the terrain concerning people with intellectual disabilities before we begin to discuss health inequalities and public health approaches to the health of people with intellectual disabilities in the following chapters. We begin by outlining the major ways in which the construct of intellectual disability has been understood and operationalised, and discuss the implications of these different ways of understanding intellectual disability for how the health inequalities experienced by people with intellectual disabilities are to be understood and addressed. We describe the major issues concerned with identifying and classifying intellectual disability, followed by an overview of the research concerning the epidemiology and causes of intellectual disabilities.

Understanding intellectual disability

Frameworks for understanding disability in general and intellectual disability in particular are constantly developing and hotly contested (Buntinx and Schalock, 2010; Officer and Groce, 2009; Open Society Institute, 2006; Thomas, 2007). It is important to sketch out how different frameworks conceptualise intellectual disability, as they have very different implications for how we understand the health inequalities experienced by people with intellectual disabilities and what can and should be done about them.

The medical model

Within high-income countries (and within some low- and middle-income countries too; see Emerson, Fujiura and Hatton, 2007), the dominant framework for understanding disability in the last 100 years has been what has been described as the 'medical' or 'individual' model (World Health Organization, 2001). This characterises the inequalities experienced by people with intellectual disabilities (for example in the areas of work or health) as an inevitable function of the long-standing 'deficits' located within individuals. In this model, the duty of society is to work towards the eradication or prevention of the conditions 'causing' intellectual disabilities (for example, through genetic screening programmes), to work on rehabilitating individuals to reduce the magnitude of their 'deficits', and to 'care' for this section of the population in comfortable conditions. Notions of striving for social justice through notions of social equality do not apply here as they are viewed as unrealistic, unachievable and irrelevant to the societal tasks at hand.

The social model

In explicit contrast to the medical model is the social model of disability (Stalker, 2012; Thomas, 2007). The social model makes a conceptual distinction between *impairment* (an injury, illness or condition that is associated with long-term differences and/or limitations in potential functioning) and *disability* (the economic, social, physical and cultural barriers that exclude people with impairments from fully participating in society as equal citizens). This model characterises the inequalities experienced by people with intellectual disabilities as the expression of societal oppression and exclusion rather than being the inevitable consequence of a person's impairment. Therefore political action is required to eradicate the economic, social, physical and cultural structures and processes that oppress people with intellectual disabilities, and to ensure that human rights are afforded to people with intellectual disabilities (Barnes, 2012). It is important to note that the social model is primarily a framework for political change rather than a fully elaborated theory (Barnes, 2012), and there are current debates about the importance or otherwise of recognising the 'reality' of impairments and the direct and indirect effects they may have on a person's health and well-being (Stalker, 2012; Thomas, 2007).

The biopsychosocial model

Various attempts have been made to reconcile the medical and social models, the most influential of which is the International Classification of Functioning, Disability and Health (ICF) developed by the World Health Organization (World Health Organization, 2001, 2007b). Despite the medical and social models being in explicit conflict with each other, the ICF 'is based on an integration of these two opposing models' (World Health Organization, 2001; p.20).

In the ICF, functioning and disability are conceptualised in terms of the complex interplay between bodily functions/structures (and the immediate impairment effects of these), activities (and activity limitations), participation (and participation restrictions) and environmental factors. Environmental factors (such as living conditions, social attitudes and practices, service systems and policies) are explicitly recognised as having a crucial effect on a person's functioning and social participation (or social inclusion). As such, disability arises when people with impairments are confronted by social conditions (or environmental barriers) that reduce their everyday activities and/or social participation (World Health Organization, 2001). Disability is not seen as a characteristic of a person.

Neither is it seen as an inevitable consequence of a particular disease or health condition. Rather, it is viewed as a socially determined outcome resulting from the operation of disabling and discriminatory cultural, social and environmental conditions.

The ambition of the ICF is to create an overarching framework, or 'language', within which the full complexity of disabled people's lives can be captured and classified. However, in spirit and operation the ICF can resemble a medical model on to which social model aspects have been grafted. For example, the construct of human rights is not an integral part of the ICF framework (Bickenbach, 2012). Furthermore, the very complexity of the ICF does not readily lend itself to the identification of clear priorities for identifying and eliminating the inequalities experienced by people with intellectual disabilities.

Mapping models of intellectual disability on to health and health inequalities

The models outlined above clearly conceptualise intellectual disability very differently, with very different actions recommended as a consequence. What do these models of disability have to say about health and health inequalities?

The medical model of disability is consistent with (and possibly arose from) a bio-medical model of health. Health is conceptualised as the absence of disease, where disease is created by physical causal agents (genes, bio-chemicals, damage to the body) leading to changes in the structure and function of the physical body and brain, with interventions (typically medication or surgery) directed to these physical agents. Because the medical model views intellectual disability itself as a series of functional deficits caused by physical causal agents, this model in effect fuses the constructs of impairment, disability and poor health/disease. For the medical model, reducing the health inequalities experienced by people with intel-lectual disabilities compared to others in society is an irrelevant goal – the goal is to reduce the poor health experienced by people with intellectual disabilities who will, however, always remain in poorer health than the general population.

The social model of disability views health inequalities as one expression or indicator of the oppressive ways in which societies treat people with intellec-tual disabilities. Although this is becoming increasingly contested (Barnes, 2012; Shakespeare, 2006), the social model makes clear conceptual distinctions between impairment, disability and health. An impairment is not inevitably equivalent to poor health or illness, although there is increasing discussion amongst disability studies theorists that there can be direct 'impairment effects', which have an impact on health (Scambler, 2012; Shakespeare, 2006; Thomas, 2007). Whilst the political action required by the social model to achieve equal civil rights and empowerment includes eliminating inequities in access to effective health services and changing societies to eliminate the disablism that can result in poorer health and well-being, achieving civil rights and empowerment would be the primary goal of the social model.

The biopsychosocial model of disability is consistent with a more holistic conception of health, such as that adopted by the World Health Organization: 'Health is a state of complete physical, mental, and social well-being and not merely the absence of disease or infirmity' (World Health Organization, 1946). This definition emphasises health as positive well-being within a broad social context, rather than health as being the absence of disease within an individual. Using this holistic conception of health means that good health or poor health are distributed across the components of the ICF in terms of how bodily functions/structures (and the immediate impairment effects of these), activities (and activity limitations), participation (and participation restrictions) and environmental factors interact (Buntinx and Schalock, 2010). Biopsychosocial frameworks such as the ICF certainly allow for the identification of health inequalities (and would identify a much broader range of inequalities as falling within the 'health' domain compared with the medical model). The ICF, however, is studiously neutral on what the ultimate goals of policy and practice concerning the health of people with intellectual disabilities should be, and what the priorities are for achieving them.

The capabilities framework

An increasingly influential framework for documenting, understanding and addressing inequalities in society is the capabilities (or capability) framework (Nussbaum, 2011; Sen, 2001). The capabilities framework has arisen out of work on the economics of developing countries, with an original ambition to move beyond a country's Gross Domestic Product (GDP) as an indicator of how 'well' a country is developing. As many authors have pointed out (Nussbaum, 2011; Sen, 2001; Wilkinson, 2005; Wilkinson and Pickett, 2009), a nation with higher or rapidly increasing GDP can also be a nation with huge levels of inequality that suppresses the rights of its citizens.

The capabilities framework (or more properly frameworks, as its most high-profile proponents disagree on many aspects of the framework) has a number of characteristics that make it an encouraging approach for understanding the health and other inequalities experienced by people with intellectual disabilities and prioritising societal action to address these health inequalities. Still in development, there is increasing recognition that a capabilities framework may have substantial utility for disabled people generally (Burchardt, 2004; Wolff, 2011), including people with cognitive impairments (Nussbaum, 2009; Wolff, 2009).

As Nussbaum (2011) describes the central focus of a capabilities approach:

- The key question to ask, when comparing societies and assessing them for their basic decency or justice, is, 'What is each person able to do and to be?' In other words, the approach takes *each person as an end*, asking not just about the total or average well-being but about the opportunities available to each person.

- It is *focused on choice or freedom*, holding that the crucial good societies should be promoting for their people is a set of opportunities, or substantial freedoms, which people then may or may not exercise in action: the choice is theirs. It thus commits itself to respect for people's powers of self-definition.
- The approach is resolutely *pluralist about value*: it holds that the capability achievements that are central for people are different in quality, not just in quantity; that they cannot without distortion be reduced to a single numerical scale; and that a fundamental part of understanding and producing them is understanding the specific nature of each.
- Finally, the approach is *concerned with entrenched social injustice and inequality*, especially capability failures that are the result of discrimination or marginalization. It ascribes an urgent *task to government and public policy* – namely, to improve the quality of life for all people, as defined by their capabilities (pp. 18–19; italics in the original).

It is important to note that capabilities are not synonymous with skills or abilities. For Nussbaum (2011), capabilities 'are not just abilities residing inside a person but also the freedoms or opportunities created by a combination of personal abilities and the political, social, and economic environment' (p. 20). Nussbaum calls these *substantial freedoms* or *combined capabilities*, as meaningfully exercising these capabilities requires both *internal capabilities* (states of the person amenable to change, including learned skills but also states such as self-confidence) and the *social, political and economic conditions* in which people can develop and apply their internal capabilities.

These combined capabilities are conceptually distinct from people's *basic capabilities* (the 'innate equipment' that makes development possible). Because capability frameworks are focused on 'What is each person able to do and to be?' in terms of freedoms for each and every individual, no minimum threshold of basic capabilities is required and no one is excluded on grounds of cognitive impairment from the responsibilities of societies to facilitate the individual exercise of combined capabilities (Nussbaum, 2009; Wolff, 2009).

Combined capabilities are also conceptually distinct from *functioning* (how capabilities are realised in people's lives). The exercise of self-determination via combined capabilities will result in different people choosing different ways of living their lives.

The capabilities framework and health inequalities

To make this rather abstract discussion more concrete, we will take as an example the inequalities in physical activity levels experienced by people with intellectual disabilities (Bartlo and Klein, 2011; Robertson et al., 2000b) and discuss how different models approach this issue.

The capabilities framework is centrally concerned with ensuring that each and every person with intellectual disabilities has the combined capabilities to exercise self-determination in terms of physical activity. This would include ensuring that a person has been supported to develop relevant internal capabilities, such as knowledge about the health and other consequences of physical activity or inactivity, and self-efficacy in terms of perceived control over levels and types of physical activity. It would also include the person living throughout their life in environments that actively support and do not hinder the exercise of self-determination in relation to physical activity. For children, this may include local schools that facilitate a wide range of sports and other physical activities that would be accessible and potentially enjoyable to the person, interpersonal environments free of bullying or negative reactions to the person engaging in physical activity, and anti-poverty social policies to support families in facilitating physical activity for their children.

For the capabilities framework, the aim is for people with intellectual disabilities to be able to exercise substantial freedoms in terms of physical activity. Different people may make different choices in terms of the level and type of physical activity (so their functionings may be quite different), but it is crucial that they have not made these choices due to the curtailed development of their internal capabilities or unsupportive environments. It is also important to note that a person's basic capabilities will have an influence on how their combined capabilities are to be achieved (for example for a person in a wheelchair compared with an ambulant person), but the duty of societies aiming for social justice is to achieve combined capabilities for all people with intellectual disabilities.

This example highlights some of the strengths and challenges of the capabilities framework as applied to the health inequalities of people with intellectual disabilities.

First, there is a question about what we should measure to determine whether people with intellectual disabilities are living in a just society with regard to health. Some capability framework theorists argue that it is the combined capabilities or substantial freedoms that are crucial (Nussbaum, 2011) – that people with intellectual disabilities are in a position to genuinely exercise substantial freedom with regard to their health. This places capability frameworks firmly in line with human rights frameworks (Burchardt, 2008), where human rights can be seen as another way of describing important domains of substantial freedoms. It also means that capability frameworks are not compatible with quality of life approaches to evaluating the lives of people with intellectual disabilities, with their emphasis on assessing quality of life in hedonic and materialist terms (Hatton, 1998; Buntinx and Schalock, 2010). However, direct assessment and measurement of substantial freedoms (as with human rights) is notoriously difficult (Wolff, 2011).

Other authors using capability frameworks argue that we can see whether substantial freedoms are being exercised through the functionings that result from the combined capabilities that people have at their disposal (Wolff, 2011; Wolff and De-Shalit, 2007). This might be particularly relevant to the health of people with intellectual disabilities, where stark inequalities in functionings related to health are clearly visible. However, even if health functionings are taken as the end point, it is still crucial within a capability framework to understand how these inequalities in health functionings have arisen (particularly by investigating people's internal capabilities and the social, political and economic conditions within which they live) to inform societal action. An attempt to operationalise a capabilities framework within a UK policy context recommends assessing capabilities in terms of autonomy, treatment (both aspects of substantial freedoms) and functionings (Burchardt and Vizard, 2011).

Second, capability frameworks are concerned with social justice as it applies to each and every individual, rather than an approach that is concerned only with inequality at an aggregate level (Wolff and De-Shalit, 2007). In terms of addressing the health inequalities of people with intellectual disabilities, this would not necessarily mean ensuring that the health functionings (or the combined capabilities) of this group as a whole were similar to those of the general population – a stated goal of many policies designed to reduce or eliminate health inequalities. Instead, it would mean ensuring that each and every person with intellectual disabilities met or exceeded minimum thresholds in terms of health functionings (Nussbaum, 2011). Achieving population equality would be inadequate if some people with intellectual disabilities did not meet minimum thresholds in terms of health, although there is debate about how such minimum thresholds should be set and whether they should be absolute or relative, for example when considering hardship and poverty (Wolff and De-Shalit, 2007). Of course, assessing health inequalities between people with intellectual disabilities and the rest of the population is important for understanding the scale and nature of disadvantage experienced by people with intellectual disabilities but, according to the capability framework, eliminating health inequalities is not necessarily the ultimate goal of social policy.

A third characteristic of capability frameworks is that they are pluralist about value – in other words, every domain of combined capabilities (or possibly functionings) is important in its own right, rather than being reducible to a single scale (Nussbaum, 2011). For example, both access to effective cancer screening services and healthy levels of physical activity are important for people with intellectual disabilities to experience, and achieving exceptional levels of physical activity would not absolve society of responsibility for accessible cancer screening services just because a pooled measure of 'health' averaging across these domains might turn out as satisfactory. In this sense it is clearly in opposition to quality of life approaches to assessing the lives of people with intellectual disabilities (Buntinx and Schalock, 2010), which explicitly include the facility to combine domain scores into a single quality of life index score for an individual. It also makes clear that there may be trade-offs or 'tragic choices' to be made between different capabilities in certain circumstances (Nussbaum, 2011): for example, the family of a child with intellectual disabilities may feel they have to make a trade-off between their child attending a segregated school and the child receiving no education at all if no inclusive education is available to their child.

Finally, additions to capabilities frameworks have highlighted additional concepts of potential value when understanding the health inequalities experienced by people with intellectual disabilities. This includes the concept of 'capability security' – individuals feeling secure that societies will not withdraw the supports and conditions essential to the achievement of substantial freedoms (Wolff and De-Shalit, 2007). For example, people with intellectual disabilities and their families may feel considerable anxiety about benefits and/or services being withdrawn, reducing the potential positive impact that they could make of current benefits and services (Wilkinson, 2005; Wolff, 2011). The same authors (Wolff and De-Shalit, 2007) also discuss the concept of 'fertile functioning' where one area of capability may promote others (for example, people with intellectual disabilities who are physically active may also be more socially connected and able to access employment), and the concept of 'corrosive disadvantage' where one area of unmet capability may block others (for example, people with intellectual disabilities who are depressed are blocked from enjoying a whole range of substantial freedoms in other domains).

Taken together, these central features of capability frameworks provide a potentially coherent and useful way of both understanding the health inequalities of people with intellectual disabilities and guiding public policy towards improving the public health of this group. A capability framework is compatible with the social model of disability, embedding the central insights of the social model within a broader conceptual framework without losing the political importance of striving for social justice (Burchardt, 2004). It is also compatible with human rights approaches, again embedding human rights within a broader conceptual framework whilst retaining the importance of individual and indivisible human rights (Burchardt and Vizard, 2011). In contrast with both the medical model and the ICF, capability frameworks are explicitly concerned with social justice and the responsibility of societies to ensure that each and every individual is in a position to exercise substantial freedoms. The emphasis on the importance of each dimension of substantial freedoms and on these freedoms themselves also makes capability frameworks incompatible with quality-of-life approaches.

Which capabilities are important?

An essential part of the capabilities framework is trying to determine which capabilities are the central ones for people with intellectual disabilities, with capability theorists taking different approaches. Nussbaum (2011) has developed ten 'central capabilities' from a priori philosophical principles, which she argues apply to all humans. In contrast, Sen (1999) argues that central capabilities should be determined democratically in response to societal concerns, although he does recognise that this may lead to capabilities that are 'trivial' or even 'bad'. Hybrid approaches have also been tried; these start with a set of capabilities derived from human rights principles then empirically develop these capabilities through processes of deliberative consultation (Burchardt and Vizard, 2011; Wolff and De-Shalit, 2007).

As far as we are aware, the development of a specific set of central capabilities for people with intellectual disabilities has not been attempted, although there has been a substantial international research effort to develop quality-of-life domains for disabled people generally (Power, Green and Grp, 2010) and people with intellectual disabilities in particular (Wang et al., 2010; Claes et al., 2010), and a set of central human rights for disabled people has also been developed (United Nations, 2006b).

Table 1.1 below presents an initial attempt at a crosswalk comparing the central domains of life proposed in: (1) quality-of-life models for people with intellectual disabilities and disabled people generally; (2) the UN Convention on the rights of persons with disabilities; (3) Nussbaum's ten central capabilities; and (4) the 'valuable capabilities' developed partly empirically with members of the public in the UK. This definitively non-definitive crosswalk aims to comparatively map the major central domains of life as described by each approach, although many of the major central domains (and particularly the sub-domains described as constituting them) are described and grouped in ways that make this difficult.

Nevertheless, there is considerable consistency across these approaches, particularly at the level of sub-domains. For our purposes, there is a clear recognition across all the approaches of the importance of good health, in terms of not dying prematurely and experiencing good bodily health and emotional well-being. Despite differing emphases, there are also considerable commonalities in other central domains of life that could be considered as the internal capabilities and social, political and economic conditions that facilitate good health, such as good interpersonal relationships, legal security and equality before the law, material well-being, inclusion as a full member of society, having a productive role in society, and being supported to achieve substantial freedoms in terms of knowledge, skills and the capacity for meaningful self-determination. These broader factors that facilitate (or hinder) the exercise of substantial freedoms in terms of health are as much of a concern as access to effective health services for those seeking to improve the health of people with intellectual disabilities.

A recent attempt to operationalise central capabilities within a UK policy context, building on the ten 'valuable capabilities', suggests the adoption of 'spotlight indicators' (Alkire et al., 2009; Burchardt and Vizard, 2011). These are pragmatic, in that they are typically based on statistics already being collected, and they are not designed to be comprehensive across all aspects of the valuable capabilities or across the three aspects of capabilities they propose to assess (autonomy, treatment and functionings). Potential spotlight indicators for England that directly assess health capabilities and that are potentially relevant to people with intellectual disabilities are listed in Table 1.2. However, it should be noted that almost all the other spotlight indicators can be considered as either internal capabilities of the person or aspects of the person's social, economic and political conditions, all of which will have a profound effect on the person's autonomy, treatment and functionings in relation to health.

Table 1.1 Central domains of experience according to: (1) quality-of-life framework for people with intellectual disabilities; (2) World Health Organization (WHO) quality-of-life framework including a disability module; (3) UN Convention on the Rights of Persons with Disabilities; (4) the 'central capabilities' derived by Nussbaum from fundamental principles; and (5) the 'valuable capabilities' developed for the Equality and Human Rights Commission (EHCR) on the basis of codified human rights and a deliberative consultation process

Central domains of life (with sub-domains) according to each approach

QoL for people with intellectual disabilities (Wang et al., 2010; Claes et al., 2010)	WHO QoL including disability module (Power et al., 2010)	UN Convention on the Rights of Persons with Disabilities (United Nations, 2006)	'Central capabilities' (Nussbaum, 2011)	'Valuable capabilities' (Burchardt, 2008; Burchardt and Vizard, 2011)
Overall QoL derived from combining subjective and objective QoL scores in each sub-domain	Overall QoL (separate item)			
Physical well-being, health (functioning, symptoms, fitness, nutrition)	General health	Article 10: Right to life	Life: Being able to live to the end of a human life of normal length	Life
Activities of daily living (self-care, mobility)	Physical health (pain, medication, energy, mobility, sleep, ADS, work)	Article 15: Freedom from torture or cruel, inhuman or degrading treatment or punishment	Not dying prematurely, or before one's life is so reduced as to be not worth living	Health
Healthcare	Psychological health (positive feelings, spirituality, thinking, body image, self-esteem, negative feelings)	Article 16: Freedom from exploitation, violence and abuse	Bodily health:	Bodily integrity
Leisure (recreation, hobbies)		Article 17: Right to respect for physical and mental integrity	Being able to have good health, including reproductive health	
			To be adequately nourished	

To have adequate shelter

Play:
Being able to laugh, to play, to enjoy recreational activities

Article 20: Right to personal mobility through provision of affordable aids, equipment, assistive technology and personal support

Article 25: Right to healthcare and early identification and intervention without discrimination

Article 30: Right to participation in cultural life, recreation, leisure and sport

Emotions:
Being able to have attachments to things and people outside oneself

To love those who love and care for one, to grieve at their absence

In general, to love, to grieve, to experience longing, gratitude and justified anger

Not having one's emotional development blighted by fear and anxiety

Emotional well-being
Contentment (satisfaction, moods, enjoyment)
Self-concept (identity, self-worth, self-esteem)
Lack of stress (predictability and control)

Table 1.1 (cont.)

Central domains of life (with sub-domains) according to each approach

Interpersonal relations Interactions (social networks, social contacts) Relationship (family, friends, peers) Support (emotional, physical, financial)	Social (personal relationships, sexual activity, social support)	Article 23: Right to non-discrimination in all matters relating to marriage, family, parenthood, relationships and fertility	Affiliation: Being able to live with and towards others, to recognise and show concern for other human beings, to engage in various forms of social interaction, to be able to imagine the situation of another Having the social bases of self-respect and nonhumiliation Being able to be treated as a dignified being whose worth is equal to that of others	Individual, family and social life
Rights Human (respect, dignity, equality) Legal (citizenship, access, due process)	Disabilities module (impact of disability, discrimination, advocacy, future prospects, control, choice, autonomy; communication ability, social acceptance, respect, social network and interaction)	Article 5: Equality before the law and non-discrimination Article 8: Right to have states parties raise awareness, combat prejudices and foster respect for the rights and dignity of persons with disabilities	Bodily integrity: Being able to move freely from place to place To be secure against violent assault, including sexual assault and domestic violence Having opportunities for sexual satisfaction and for choice in matters of reproduction	Legal security

Article 12: Right to equal recognition before the law and legal capacity on an equal basis with others

Article 13: Equal access to justice

Article 14: Right to liberty and security of the person

Article 18: Freedom of movement and nationality

Article 22: Respect for privacy regardless of place of residence or living arrangements

Article 29: Right to participate as equals in political and public life

Control over one's environment:

Political. Being able to participate effectively in political choices that govern one's life; having the right of political participation, and protections of free speech and association

Material. Being able to hold property (both land and movable goods) and having property rights on an equal basis with others; having the right to seek employment on an equal basis with others; having the freedom from unwarranted search and seizure

In work, being able to work as a human being, exercising practical reason and entering into meaningful relationships of mutual recognition with other workers

Table 1.1 (*cont.*)

Central domains of life (with sub-domains) according to each approach

Material well-being Financial status (income, benefits) Employment (work status, work environment) Housing (type of residence, ownership)	Article 9: Equal access to the physical environment, transportation, information and communications Article 27: Right to work on an equal basis with others Article 28: Right to an adequate standard of living and social protection		Adequate standard of living
Social inclusion Community integration and participation Community roles (contributor, volunteer) Social supports (support networks, services)	Article 19: Right to live and participate in the community		Participation, influence and voice
Self-determination Autonomy/personal control (independence) Goals and personal values (desires, expectations) Choices (opportunities, options, preferences)	Article 21: Freedom of expression and opinion, and equal access to information	Practical reason: Being able to form a conception of the good and to engage in critical reflection about the planning of one's life	Identity, expression and self-respect

Education and learning

Personal development
Education (achievements, education status)
Personal competence (cognitive, social, practical)

Article 24: Right to education within the general education system, without discrimination
Article 26: Right to habilitation and rehabilitation services in order to attain and maintain maximum independence

Senses, imagination and thought
Being able to use the senses, to imagine, think and reason – and to do these things in a way informed and cultivated by an adequate education
Being able to use imagination and thought in connection with experiencing and producing works and events of one's own choice, religious, literary, musical and so forth
Being able to use one's mind in ways protected by guarantees of freedom of expression with respect to both political and artistic speech, and freedom of religious exercise
Being able to have pleasurable experiences and to avoid non-beneficial pain

Table 1.1 (*cont.*)

Central domains of life (with sub-domains) according to each approach

Performance (success, achievement, productivity)		Productive and valued activities
	Other species: Being able to live with concern for and in relation to animals, plants and the world of nature	

Table 1.2 Spotlight indicators that could directly assess the health capabilities of people with intellectual disabilities (Alkire et al., 2009)

A. LIFE
Indicator 1: Life expectancy
1.1: Period life expectancy at birth, and ages 20, 65 and 80
Indicator 2: Homicide
2.1: Homicide rate
Indicator 3: Other specific-cause mortality rates
3.1: Cardiovascular disease mortality rate (age-standardised)
3.2: Cancer mortality rate (age-standardised)
3.3: Suicide rate
3.4: Accident mortality rate
Indicator 4: Death rates from non-natural causes for people resident or detained in public or private institutions
4.3: Deaths from non-natural causes for people resident or detained in health or social care establishments

B. HEALTH
Indicator 1: Limiting illness, disability and mental health
1.1: Percentage who report a long-standing health problem or disability that substantially limits their ability to carry out normal day-to-day activities
1.2: Percentage who report poor mental health and well-being
Indicator 2: Subjective evaluation of current health status
2.1: Percentage who report poor current health status
Indicator 3: Dignity and respect in health treatment
3.1: Percentage with low perceptions of treatment with dignity and respect in healthcare
3.2: Percentage reporting lack of support for individual nutritional needs during hospital stays
Indicator 4: Healthy living
4.1: Percentage who are living a healthy lifestyle, covering (a) smoking (b) alcohol (c) physical activity (d) consumption of fruit and vegetables (e) body mass
4.2: Percentage who are living in an area with less favourable environmental conditions
Indicator 5: Vulnerability to accidents
5.1: Accident and Emergency accident and injury rate, by location

F. STANDARD OF LIVING
Indicator 3: Access to care
3.1: Percentage of disabled people (including older people) who do not receive practical support that meets their needs
Indicator 4: Quality of the local area
4.1: Percentage living in an area with 'unsatisfactory' or 'poor' local environmental conditions
Indicator 5: Being treated with respect by private companies and public agencies in relation to your standard of living
5.1: Percentage who report being treated unfairly by financial institutions, utility companies, housing officials or private landlords, social services, Jobcentre Plus or the Pension Service, or who have avoided contacting them for fear of being treated unfairly

Classifying intellectual disabilities

When investigating the scale and nature of the health inequalities experienced by people with intellectual disabilities in public health or population terms, a crucial foundation stone is identifying which people can be considered to have an intellectual disability.

In high-income countries, the 'gold standard' classification system for identifying people with intellectual disabilities is often seen as that provided by the American Association on Intellectual and Developmental Disabilities, with the following definition: 'Intellectual disability is characterized by significant limitations both in intellectual functioning and in adaptive behaviour as expressed in conceptual, social, and practical adaptive skills. This disability originates before age 18' (AAIDD, 2010):

- A significant limitation in intellectual functioning is operationalised as 'an IQ score that is approximately two standard deviations below the mean (typically 70–75), considering the standard error of measurement for the specific assessment instruments used and the instruments' strengths and limitations'.
- A significant limitation in adaptive behaviour is operationalised as 'performance on a standardized measure of adaptive behavior that is normed on the general population including people with and without ID that is approximately two standard deviations below the mean of either (a) one of the following three types of adaptive behavior; conceptual, social, and practical or (b) an overall score on a standardized measure of conceptual, social, and practical skills'.
- The age 18 threshold is used because a person's 18th birthday approximates the age in US society that a person typically assumes adult roles, and is partly used to distinguish people with intellectual disabilities from people who acquire or develop intellectual impairments after they have become an adult (e.g. through acquired brain injuries or dementia).

However, the discussion in the previous section about how different models consider intellectual disability begins to illustrate how fraught such an apparently straightforward method for identification is. Methods for identifying and classifying people with intellectual disabilities inevitably rest upon assumptions about the nature of intellectual disability, all of which are open to debate.

First, there is the question of what 'intellectual' means in the context of intellectual disabilities. Within classification systems such as the one outlined above (AAIDD, 2010), intellectual functioning is assumed to be a unitary construct that can be assessed quantitatively (typically by using IQ tests). The validity of IQ tests has been vigorously contested, with better IQ test performance robustly associated with the nature and duration of experience of formal education, familiarity with the type of stimuli used in IQ tests, and socialisation into the situation of being tested (Flynn, 1987). Because of socio-economic differences between ethnic groups within high-income societies, this can result in considerable over-identification of intellectual disabilities amongst minority ethnic communities (Hatton, 2002; Leonard and Wen, 2002). There have also been more fundamental challenges to the construct of unitary intelligence from a cross-cultural perspective (Sternberg, 1997), with intelligence not considered to be a universally valid construct that is easily separable from the cultural contexts within which people live.

Second, should the identification of intellectual disability be concerned with intellectual impairment (in capability theory terms, a set of basic capabilities) or with the disability associated with intellectual impairment that people experience (in capability theory terms, a set of internal capabilities)? Although intelligence tests are theoretically designed to test a set of basic capabilities, their context-dependent nature and amenability to learning/practice effects (Flynn, 1987) suggest that they are actually assessing a set of internal capabilities. Furthermore, there has been a long-standing recognition in classification systems that assessing intellectual impairment is insufficient to identify whether a person is intellectually disabled (AAIDD, 2010) – in other words, intellectual impairment does not determine the internal capabilities of a person in terms of the skills and behaviours they actually exercise in their day-to-day lives. To this end, classification systems also measure the 'adaptive behaviours' (for example, functional numeracy in terms of telling the time or being able to use and understand money) that people display in their day-to-day lives (AAIDD, 2010).

Taken together, the focus in classification systems on internal capabilities rather than notional basic capabilities means that intellectual disability is a profoundly social construct (Stalker, 2012) – it is a snapshot of what a society has allowed a person to make of their basic capabilities in the environment within which they live at a particular point in time. With a different personal history and in a different environment, these internal capabilities could be very different, such that it is possible that a person could move back and forth between being classified as intellectually disabled or not. It is certainly the case that who counts as having an 'intellectual disability' has varied hugely over time (Wright and Digby, 1996; Trent, 1994), and across cultures and countries (Emerson et al., 2007; Jenkins, 1998).

The epidemiology of intellectual disabilities

The ineluctably social nature of intellectual disability presents a profound challenge to the methods used by epidemiologists to investigate intellectual disabilities. Epidemiology has been defined as 'the study of the distribution and determinants of health, disease, and disorder in human populations' (Fryers, 1993). Although intellectual disability is neither a disease nor a disorder, a public health approach to people with intellectual disabilities is greatly assisted by evidence concerning the *incidence* (the number of new cases arising in a population in a stated period of time) and *prevalence* (the number of cases, old and new, existing in a population at a given point in time or over a specified period) of intellectual disabilities, and the social, cultural, economic and environmental conditions that are associated with incidence and prevalence.

In practice, most epidemiological research concerning the incidence or prevalence of intellectual disabilities, particularly in high-income countries, has simply used an IQ threshold alone to classify whether a person has an intellectual disability, although the addition of adaptive behaviours may make little difference to prevalence estimates (Obi et al., 2011). This strand of research has also typically used bands of IQ scores to classify 'levels' of intellectual disability, most commonly making a distinction between 'mild' intellectual disability (IQ 50–70) and 'severe' intellectual disability (IQ <50).

Incidence

Epidemiological studies of the incidence of intellectual disability are relatively scarce, largely due to their methodological difficulty (Durkin, 2002; Fryers, 1993). These studies tend to rely on administratively defined populations of people with intellectual disabilities (typically people identified as such by service systems) rather than independently assessing entire populations, resulting in possible under-estimates of incidence for people with mild intellectual disabilities. Studies across the USA and Northern Europe have reported similar incidence rates – for example, a US study reported a cumulative incidence at age 8 years of 4.9 children with severe intellectual disabilities per 1000 births, and 4.3 children with mild intellectual disabilities per 1000 births (Katusic et al., 1995; Rantakallio and von Wendt, 1986).

Even less epidemiological evidence is available concerning the incidence of intellectual disabilities in low- and middle-income countries (Durkin, 2002; World Health Organization, 2007a). There are, however, very plausible reasons to suggest that exposure to potential *environmental* causes of intellectual disabilities is likely to show substantial regional and international variation, thereby leading to variations in incidence, with higher incidence likely amongst poorer low- and middle-income countries compared with high-income countries (World Health Organization, 2011b).

Prevalence

Epidemiological studies of the prevalence of intellectual disabilities of children and adults across the world's high-income countries are becoming more common (Leonard and Wen, 2002; Maulik et al., 2011; Roeleveld, Zielhuis and Gabreels, 1997). Prevalence estimates for the world's middle- and low-income countries are more sparse and varied for a number of reasons, but are increasing in number and geographical scope (Maulik et al., 2011). In a global context, it is important to remember that the construct of intellectual disability itself is highly context-dependent and possibly culture-specific (Emerson et al., 2007). Anthropological work suggests that all societies may make distinctions between competent and incompetent people, with competence broadly defined as 'the capacity or potential for adequate functioning-in-context as a socialised human' (Jenkins, 1998), although there seems to be little consistency across societies in what counts as competent or incompetent (Jenkins, 1998).

A recent meta-analysis of 52 studies estimating the prevalence of intellectual disability from around the world (Maulik et al., 2011) calculated an overall prevalence rate of intellectual disability of 10.37 people per 1000 population. The number of studies included in the meta-analysis allowed the authors to investigate factors associated with variations in reported prevalence rates across studies, although, because many of these factors co-vary with each other, it is impossible to determine their relative importance in determining variation in prevalence rates. For example, studies in high-income countries (associated with lower prevalence rates) are also more likely to conduct studies on a wider geographical basis and identify people using standard diagnostic or intellectual disability criteria (also associated with lower prevalence rates). Factors associated with variations in prevalence rates include:

- Gender – intellectual disability was more common in both male children and adults compared with female children and adults, although female-to-male ratios varied across studies (0.7–0.9 for children/adolescents; 0.4–1.0 for adults).
- Age – studies reporting prevalence rates for children/adolescents tended to report higher prevalence rates (18.30/1000) than studies focusing on adults (4.94/1000). This might partly be due to more comprehensive identification of intellectual disability in education systems compared with later in adulthood, and may also partly be the consequence of differential mortality throughout adulthood.
- Income group of countries – studies in low-income countries reported the highest prevalence rates (16.41/1000), followed by middle-income countries (15.94/1000) and high-income countries (9.21/1000).
- Type of population – studies working in rural areas (19.88/1000) or urban slums/mixed rural–urban areas (21.23/1000) reported higher prevalence rates compared with studies working in larger regional/provincial areas (7.85/1000).
- Sampling strategy – studies that used random household survey samples reported higher prevalence rates (15.78/1000) than those using administratively defined populations (i.e. those currently using services for people with intellectual disabilities or those known to services) (9.35/1000).
- Study design – studies using cohort designs reported higher prevalence rates (31.21/1000) than those using cross-sectional designs (9.69/1000).
- Identification method – studies using a broad psychological assessment/screening tool reported higher prevalence rates (14.30/1000) than those applying either general psychiatric diagnostic criteria (8.68/1000) or disability-specific criteria (6.41/1000).

Although this meta-analysis could not extract data concerning 'levels' of intellectual disabilities, previous reviews of the epidemiological literature (Leonard and Wen, 2002; Roeleveld et al., 1997) largely concerning high-income countries have reported some important differences in prevalence between people with 'mild' intellectual disabilities (typically 3.7–5.9/1000, although total population studies can produce markedly higher estimates) and 'severe' intellectual disabilities (typically 3.0–4.0/1000, although total population studies can produce higher estimates).

Two other factors, largely explored within high-income countries, have been associated with increased prevalence of intellectual disabilities. The first factor concerns family ethnicity; although research is methodologically complex and different migration patterns make understanding of the findings complicated (Hatton, 2002), it does appear that certain minority ethnic communities are associated with higher prevalence rates of intellectual disabilities (Emerson, 2012a; Leonard and Wen, 2002), even when accounting for co-varying differences in socio-economic position.

The second factor contains socio-economic factors associated with gradients in the prevalence rates of intellectual disabilities. Epidemiological research has consistently reported a strong association between poorer household socio-economic position and increased prevalence rates of mild intellectual disabilities (Emerson, 2012a; Leonard and Wen, 2002; Roeleveld et al., 1997). More recently, research studies have also reported a less steep but still robust association between poorer household socio-economic position and increased prevalence rates of severe intellectual disabilities (Chapman, Scott, and Stanton-Chapman, 2008; Croen, Grether, and Selvin, 2001; Emerson, 2012a; Zheng et al., 2012).

Potential causes of intellectual disabilities

Until recently, much of the research effort concerning the identification of potential causes of intellectual disability has adopted a two-factor approach that is becoming increasingly open to debate and challenge from a public health perspective (Chapman et al., 2008; Leonard and Wen, 2002).

This two-factor approach assumed that severe intellectual disability was largely caused by bio-medical factors that were present prenatally or perinatally, and that were relatively evenly distributed across socio-economic groups. Much of the research on the causes of intellectual disability has focused on these bio-medical causes to the exclusion of investigating the social and environmental factors that may constitute 'the causes of the causes' (The Marmot Review, 2010). In contrast, mild intellectual disability was seen as largely a function of ill-defined socio-environmental factors occurring postnatally, with an inevitable association with poorer socio-economic circumstances.

More recently, the dichotomy set up by this two-factor approach has begun to dissolve under multiple challenges and has begun to be replaced by more nuanced and complex multi-factorial attempts to understand how intellectual disabilities arise (Einfeld and Emerson, 2008). First, it is clear that bio-medical causes of intellectual disabilities (such as chromosomal disorders or low birthweight) are themselves profoundly socially patterned, for example in terms of the availability and uptake of genetic screening (Louhiala, 2004) and the socio-economic factors associated with the birth of low-birthweight babies (Institute of Medicine, 2001). Second, bio-medical factors in themselves do not determine the trajectory of a person's intellectual disability (in capability framework terms, their internal capabilities) in the absence of the social, economic and environmental factors that have a profound effect on the person's intellectual development (Emerson, Hatton and Robertson, 2011d). Third, for a substantial minority (and possibly even a majority) of people with intellectual disabilities, no definite cause can be identified (Croen et al., 2001).

Most importantly, we are beginning to understand more about the social, economic and environmental factors that may interact with bio-medical factors to influence the development and maintenance of intellectual disabilities.

For example, there are a number of key environmental causes of intellectual impairments of particular significance when considering intellectual disability in both a global context and in that of developing a public health approach to minimising these causes. Key environmental causes of intellectual impairments include: transplacental infections that can occur during pregnancy (toxoplasmosis, rubella, cytomegalovirus, herpes, HIV); prenatal exposure to toxins and teratogens (e.g. alcohol, lead, mercury, maternal phenylketonuria); prenatal under-nutrition (e.g. maternal iodine deficiency); birth injury, hypoxia and rhesus incompatibility; childhood infections, especially the various types of meningitis and encephalitis; childhood exposure to environmental toxins (e.g. lead); head injury during childhood; and severe dehydration and under-nutrition (Durkin, 2002; Emerson et al., 2007).

The socio-economic gradients in the prevalence of intellectual disabilities in high-income societies outlined earlier are also beginning to be explained, in terms of processes operating throughout the child's development (Emerson et al., 2011d). *In young children*, social gradients in the prevalence of intellectual disabilities are likely to reflect two processes.

First, growing up in poverty is associated with increased exposure to a wide range of material and psychosocial hazards (e.g. preterm birth, low birth weight, foetal growth restriction, exposure to a range of toxins and teratogens, poorer nutrition including reduced rates of breast feeding, poor housing conditions, exposure to less than optimal parenting, poorer pre-school educational opportunities, injury and accidents, exposure to more hazardous neighbourhoods), all of which have been shown to impair the cognitive development of children (Andreias et al., 2010; Conger and Donnellan, 2007; Hertzman and Boyce, 2010; The Marmot Review, 2010). As a result, children exposed to 'toxic' levels of environmental adversity will be more likely than their peers to have intellectual disabilities (and in particular mild intellectual disabilities).

Second, 'selection effects' involving the intergenerational transmission of socially patterned health conditions or impairments and socio-economic position are likely to be important. For example, parents with mild intellectual disabilities are more likely than other parents to: (1) be socio-economically disadvantaged;

and (2) have a child with intellectual disabilities (IASSID Special Interest Research Group on Parents and Parenting with Intellectual Disabilities, 2008; McConnell et al., 2003; Seltzer et al., 2005).

In later childhood, it is likely that socially patterned inequalities in access to higher-quality educational activities, experiences and resources may further compromise the cognitive development of children (Andreias et al., 2010; Conger and Donnellan, 2007; Hertzman and Boyce, 2010; The Marmot Review, 2010). In capability framework terms, it is important to note how social, economic and environmental conditions 'reach back' through prenatal and perinatal causes of intellectual impairment to influence even the basic capabilities with which a child is born.

Summary

In this chapter we have attempted to reach an understanding of intellectual disability as an unavoidably social construct. We have outlined the capabilities framework and hopefully illustrated its potential utility for understanding both intellectual disability itself and the objectives of policies aiming to improve the health of people with intellectual disabilities. Finally, we have demonstrated the importance of including social, economic and environmental factors in any understanding of the development of intellectual disabilities.

Health and health inequalities

In this chapter we will define what we mean by health and then briefly discuss how the health of groups or populations is typically measured. Following this, we will define what is meant by the term health inequalities, illustrate the extent of the health inequalities that occur between and within countries, and summarise what is known about the causes of health inequalities.

Health: conceptualisation and measurement

'Health is a state of complete physical, mental, and social well-being and not merely the absence of disease or infirmity.'[1] Whilst over 65 years old, the definition of health written into the Constitution of the World Health Organization (WHO) retains its relevance in the early twenty-first century. It serves as a useful reminder that health is a positive attribute, the possession of which has implications for our physical, psychological and social well-being. As we shall see, however, the association between health and 'well-being' is far from simple.

There are four broad approaches to measuring the health of populations (e.g. the population of England) or groups within populations (e.g. people with intellectual disabilities): (1) mortality and life expectancy; (2) self-reported general health status; (3) the prevalence of specific diseases, health conditions or impairments; and (4) well-being, functioning or disability. Given that most research on health inequalities is based on the use of these measures of health, we will briefly review these approaches before discussing the definitions, scope and causes of health inequalities.

---

[1] From the Preamble to the Constitution of the World Health Organization, which entered into force on 7 April 1948.

Mortality and life expectancy

The earliest approaches to measuring the health of populations (and how this varied within populations and over time) focused on measuring the rates at which people died (mortality rates) and the age at which they died (Davey Smith, Dorling and Shaw, 2001; Kreiger, 2011). In one of the earliest examples, Louis René Villermé published a report in 1826 in which he compared annual mortality rates to the wealth of each of the twelve *arrondissements* in Paris in which people were living (Kreiger, 2011). Villermé's research indicated that, as the wealth of the *arrondissement* increased, mortality rates (risk of death within one year) systematically decreased. In 1845 Friedrich Engels, after a period working in Manchester, published his treatise on the condition of the working class in England, in which he included information on the mortality rates of people living in more or less affluent houses and in more or less affluent streets in Chorlton, an area of Manchester (Engels, 1969). In general, as both housing and neighbourhood affluence increased, risk of death decreased. Information on mortality rates for different ages can be used to calculate life expectancy (typically defined as the average number of years from birth that a person could expect to live if current trends in mortality rates were to continue for the rest of that person's life, e.g. Gillam, Yates and Badrinath, 2007).

These approaches are still used today to monitor the health of populations (and how this varies within and between populations and over time) (World Bank, 2011). Figure 2.1 illustrates variation between selected countries in infant mortality (the percentage of children dying before their first birthday) (UNICEF, 2011). The high infant mortality rates currently evident in Afghanistan (13% of children born alive dying before their first birthday) are identical to those in England and Wales in 1911 (Davey Smith et al., 2001). Figure 2.2 illustrates the change between 1990 and 2009 (in terms of difference in percentage points) in infant mortality rates for these countries (UNICEF, 2011). As can be seen, amongst poorer countries the least progress in reducing infant mortality rates has occurred in sub-Saharan Africa, with infant mortality rates actually increasing in Zimbabwe over this 20-year period. Figure 2.3 illustrates variation between these same countries in the estimated life expectancy of men and women (World Bank, 2011).

General health status

Population-based surveys and censuses commonly include a single question that asks people to rate their general health on a short scale. For example, the 2011 UK Census contained the simple question 'How is your health in general?', with possible response options being 'Very good', 'Good', 'Fair', 'Bad' and 'Very bad'. The national survey of the life experiences of adults with intellectual disabilities in England included a similar question (Emerson and Hatton, 2008c; Emerson et al., 2005). Other surveys ask parents a similar question of their children. In 2007–9, one in ten parents of seven-year-old children with intellectual disability

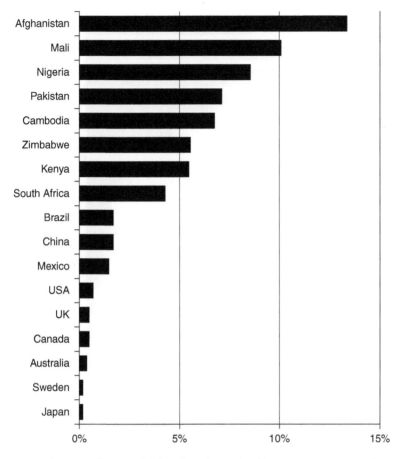

Figure 2.1 Infant mortality rates (%) by selected countries (data source: UNICEF, 2011)

in the UK rated their child's health to be 'fair' or 'poor' (rather than 'good' or 'very good') compared with one in fifty parents of children who did not have intellectual disability (Emerson et al., 2011a). Such measures are easy to collect, and predict current and future morbidity and future mortality (DeSalvo et al., 2006; Fujiura, 2012; Idler and Benyamini, 1997, 1999; Jylha, 2009).

The prevalence of specific diseases, health conditions or impairments

Whilst health is a positive attribute, many approaches to measuring the health of populations are based on measuring the prevalence of diseases, health conditions or impairments that threaten health. Two international classification systems define and categorise diseases, health conditions and impairments: the International Statistical Classification of Diseases and Related Health Problems (ICD: the

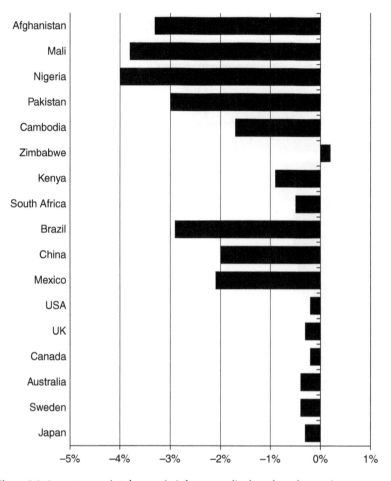

Figure 2.2 Percentage point changes in infant mortality by selected countries, 1990–2009 (data source: UNICEF, 2011)

11th revision of which is being developed at the time of writing) (World Health Organization, 2004) and the International Classification of Functioning, Disability and Health (ICF) (World Health Organization, 2001, 2007b). The primary focus of the ICD is on the classification of disease whilst the primary focus of the ICF is on the classification of human functioning and disability (Madden et al., 2012).

Prevalence refers to the proportion of the population that has a particular disease, health condition or impairment at a given point in time or over a specified period of time. Information on prevalence is typically collected either by data extraction from the administrative record systems of health services or by survey. Both methods have their strengths and weaknesses. The main strength of using data held in administrative records is that they *may* be based on detailed

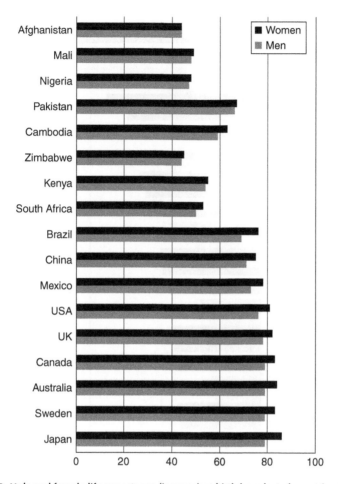

Figure 2.3 Male and female life expectancy (in years) at birth by selected countries (data source: World Bank, 2011)

clinical testing and diagnosis. Their main weakness is that they are not population based. This can be particularly problematic for estimating the prevalence of health conditions for which people will only infrequently seek treatment (e.g. common mental health problems). The main strength of survey approaches is that they can be representative of the general population (if appropriately conducted). Their main weakness is that they typically rely on people's ability to accurately self-report either that they have a particular health condition or have symptoms or signs that indicate they may have a particular health condition. Figure 2.4 uses data from the World Health Survey to illustrate the prevalence of obesity amongst people with/without disabilities across 29 European countries (Emerson et al., in press).

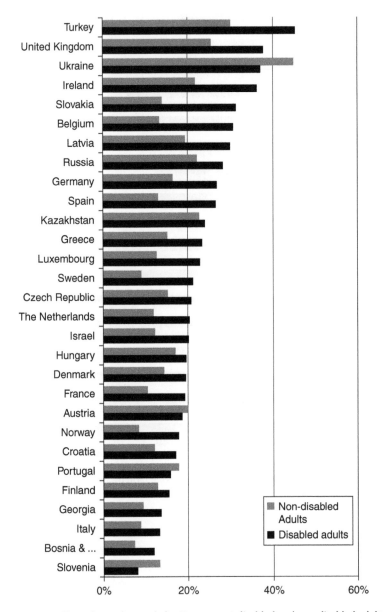

Figure 2.4 Age-adjusted prevalence of obesity amongst disabled and non-disabled adults in 29 European countries, 2002–4

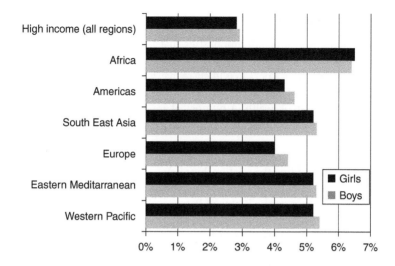

Figure 2.5 Prevalence of moderate and severe disability in children aged 0–14 years living in high-income countries and in middle- or low-income countries by WHO region using disability prevalence estimates derived from The Global Burden of Disease Estimates for 2004 (data source: World Health Organization and the World Bank, 2011)

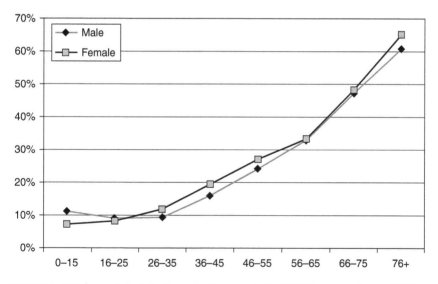

Figure 2.6 Prevalence of disability by age and gender in the UK (data source: Howe, 2010)

Functioning and disability

The WHO definition of health emphasises that health is more than 'merely the absence of disease or infirmity'. Clearly, approaches to monitoring health that are based on either how long a person is likely to live, how they perceive their health or the presence/absence of disease, health conditions or impairments cannot capture the complete meaning of health. A number of approaches have sought to provide frameworks for understanding (and potentially measuring) the impact of health on overall 'well-being'.

As noted in the previous section, the ICF seeks to provide a framework for classifying and understanding the relationships between the presence of health conditions and/or impairments and human functioning and *disability*.

The UN Convention on the Rights of Persons with Disabilities defines disability as including '… those who have long-term physical, mental, intellectual or sensory impairments which in interaction with various barriers may hinder their full and effective participation in society on an equal basis with others' (United Nations, 2006). Over the last few decades, disability has been a vigorously contested concept (Watson, Thomas and Roulstone, 2012; World Health Organization and the World Bank, 2011), with our understanding of disability moving from one in which the disadvantages experienced by people with particular health conditions or impairments were seen as the inevitable consequences of ill health (often referred to as a 'medical' or 'individual' model of disability) to one in which they are seen as being powerfully shaped by social structures and socio-cultural practices (often referred to as a 'social model' of disability) (Barnes, 2012; Shakespeare, 2006; Thomas, 2007). Within the latter framework, disability is not viewed as an inherent characteristic of individuals, but the result of the interaction between impairments and discriminatory socio-cultural practices to which people with particular health conditions or impairments may be exposed. As such, disability is being increasingly seen as a human rights issue (Hauland and Allen, 2009; Megret, 2008; United Nations, 2003, 2006; World Health Organization and the World Bank, 2011).

These changes in understanding disability are reflected (at least in part) in the ICF, in which disability is used as an 'umbrella term' to denote the negative aspects of impairments, activity limitations and participation restrictions that result from the complex interplay between health conditions and a range of personal and environmental factors (such as social attitudes and practices, services systems and policies). Measures of disability, therefore, need to take account of both the presence of a health condition or impairment and the extent to which *in that social context* the presence of a health condition or impairment is associated with limitations in activity and/or restrictions in social participation (Mont, 2007; World Health Organization and the World Bank, 2011). To date, there is little agreement on the extent or nature of limitations in activity and/or restrictions in social participation that would define disability. As a result, estimates of the prevalence of disability vary widely. Figure 2.5 illustrates the prevalence of moderate and severe disability in children living in high-income countries and in middle–low-income countries in different regions of the world, using disability prevalence estimates derived from the Global Burden of Disease estimates for 2004 (World Health Organization and the World Bank, 2011). Figure 2.6 illustrates variation in the prevalence of disability in Britain by age and gender using data extracted from the *Life Opportunities Survey* (Howe, 2010).

The value of focusing on disability as an (inverse) indicator of health is that it begins to capture something of the notion of 'physical, mental, and social well-being'. Two related approaches have sought to develop indicators of population health by combining information on life expectancy/mortality with estimates of the 'value' of life when living with a health condition, impairment or disability. Quality-adjusted life years (QALYs) combine subjective judgements about the quality of life when lived with a particular health condition, on a scale of 0 (of no value) to 1 (the same as not having that health condition), with years lived, to arrive at a measure of years lived with quality (Whitehead and Ali, 2010). Disability-adjusted life years (DALYs) combine years of life lost due to premature mortality with years of life 'lost' due to disability (Grosse et al., 2009; Murray and Lopez, 1996; World Health Organization, 2009). Again, the calculation of years of life 'lost' due to disability is based on years lived with a particular health condition and subjective judgements about the value of life when lived with a particular health condition.

Both approaches share similar ethical and conceptual problems. First, the notion that life lived with a particular health condition is of lesser 'value' runs counter to current international human rights legislation. Second, the general approach implies that the reduced value of life results from the presence of the health condition, a notion that runs counter to current approaches to understanding disability and the ICF. Third, the valuations of the quality of life when lived with a particular health condition are commonly based on judgements made by health professionals or members of the general population, who may have no direct experience of the 'value' or 'quality' of life lived with a particular health condition.

Well-being

We started the chapter with the WHO definition of health as 'not merely the absence of disease or infirmity' but 'physical, mental, and social well-being'. Nevertheless, for more than 60 years WHO has 'neither measured nor reported on well-being, focusing instead on death, disease and disability' (World Health Organization, 2013). WHO does not stand alone in its approach to measurement and reporting. Indeed, this is the norm within public health practice. But what is meant by well-being and how can we measure it?

Answering these questions is difficult but, in essence, the rather amorphous concept of well-being refers to shared cultural conceptions of people's experience of 'the good life'. Measuring well-being is a hotly contested area. Within it there are two quite distinct traditions.

The first approach is firmly rooted in attempting to understand the well-being of populations (or population sub-groups) by identifying and measuring those aspects of societal conditions that are likely to be associated with leading 'the good life' (e.g. income, education, decent housing, equality, and freedom from violence and discrimination). Typically it defines well-being as a function of life opportunities and achievements, and focuses on the objective conditions in which choices are made and that shape people's abilities to transform resources into given ends. For example, the 2009 report by the Commission on the Measurement of Economic Performance and Social Progress recommends assessing functioning and capabilities (which we discussed in Chapter 1) primarily by using objective measurement tools and indicators, but supplemented by some subjective measures (Stiglitz, Sen and Fitoussi, 2009).

The second approach defines well-being purely in terms of psychological states: 'what someone feels is what matters' (World Health Organization, 2013). A recent Organisation for Economic Co-operation and Development (OECD) review identified three separate approaches within this general area to conceptualising and measuring subjective well-being (Organisation for Economic Co-operation and Development, 2013):

- eudemonic well-being (e.g. self-perceptions of autonomy, competence, purpose of life, locus of control);
- positive and negative psychological states (e.g. the experience of joy, happiness, anxiety, sadness);
- reflective life evaluation.

Choice of approach can have significant implications with regards to: (1) their face validity when applied to policy monitoring; (2) their ability to detect between-group differences in well-being; and (3) their ability to detect changes over time in well-being as a result of government actions. With regard to face validity, as WHO has pointed out, 'in policy implementation and evaluation, governments are more easily held accountable for objective conditions [rather than subjective states]' (World Health Organization, 2013).

With regard to sensitivity, people are highly adaptive to life's changing circumstances. This is amply illustrated in the extensive evidence of the insensitivity of indicators of subjective well-being to life's changing circumstances (Diener and Biswas-Diener, 2008; Kahneman, Diener and Schwarz, 1999), a body of evidence that led to the development of set-point or homeostatic theories of subjective well-being (Brickman and Campbell, 1971; Cummins, 2003; Headey and Wearing, 1989).

This insensitivity is particularly problematic when considering the well-being of persistently marginalised or deprived groups, such as people with intellectual disabilities. As the Nobel Laureate Amartya Sen argues: 'Our desires and pleasure-taking abilities adjust to circumstances, especially to make life bearable in adverse situations ... deprived people tend to come to terms with their deprivation ... [as a result] the deprivation of the persistently deprived may look muffled and muted' (Sen, 2001).

To use indicators that may be insensitive to the scale of change that might reasonably be expected of social policy interventions could undermine the perceived value of progressive social policies (additional investment or change failing to improve subjective well-being) and inadvertently support regressive social policies (reducing the investment in or quality of supports not reducing subjective well-being). This may be particularly problematic when applied to people with intellectual disabilities, given their increased tendency to provide acquiescent responses to questions (see Chapter 3).

Take, for example, the results of the 2011/12 Personal Social Services Adult Social Care Survey in England, a national survey that included responses from 10,800 people with intellectual disabilities (The Information Centre for Health and Social Care, 2012). The survey included a general quality-of-life question: 'Thinking about all the different things in your life, good and bad, how would you say you feel about your life in general?' 81% of people with intellectual disabilities reported that their life was good or so good, it could not be any better. In comparison, only 53–7% of participants from other client groups (e.g. people with physical disabilities, people with sensory impairments) reported that their quality of life was that good. Would it be appropriate to conclude from these data that social care services in England are doing a much better job in supporting people with intellectual disabilities than other client groups? What scope do these data leave for monitoring progress? What case do they make for addressing the violations of the human rights of people with intellectual disabilities and the inadequacies of intellectual disability services in England that have been amply documented elsewhere (Care Quality Commission, 2012; House of Lords and House of Commons Joint Committee on Human Rights, 2008; Mencap, 2012a)?

Given these arguments, it is difficult not to conclude that for people with intellectual disabilities (and other persistently marginalised groups) the conceptualisation and measurement of well-being should focus on well-being within a capability framework (see Chapter 1) that views well-being as a function of life opportunities and achievements and whose measurement is best focused on the objective conditions in which people make choices and which shape their abilities to transform opportunities into their preferred ends.

Health inequalities

When measures of population health are compared across different groups, it is not uncommon to identify systematic and reliable variations in health status. The data in Figures 2.1 to 2.6 illustrate variations in different measures of health status by geographical location (country or region (2.1–2.5), gender (2.3, 2.5, 2.6), age (2.6) and disability status (2.4)). The preceding sections also contained information on the association between health and neighbourhood wealth (Villermé), housing conditions (Engels) and intellectual disability status. However, these differences in health status between groups are not necessarily health inequalities.

The term *health inequalities* refers to differences in health status between social groups 'which are unnecessary and avoidable but, in addition, are also considered unfair and unjust' (Whitehead, 1992). It is highly likely that many of the differences we have used to illustrate the preceding section of this chapter are unnecessary and avoidable and would be seen by many as also being unfair and unjust. For example, to the extent that the above differences reflect the impact of global, regional and within-country inequalities in the distribution of wealth and power, these differences are clearly unnecessary and avoidable and, hopefully to most people, unfair and unjust. But what about the shorter life expectancy of men, or of people with intellectual disabilities? To what extent are these differences unnecessary, avoidable, unfair and unjust?

The determinants of health and health inequalities

We now have nearly two centuries of research evidence that has described the association between exposure to a wide range of environmental adversities and poorer health (Adler and Stewart, 2010; Black, Morris, and Bryce, 2003; Graham, 2007; Lund et al., 2010; Marmot, 2005; Marmot and on behalf of the Commission on Social Determinants of Health, 2007; Marmot and Wilkinson, 2006; Pickett and Wilkinson, 2007; The Marmot Review, 2010; Wilkinson and Pickett, 2009; World Health Organization, 2008).

By 'environmental adversities' we are referring to a wide range of environmental material and psychosocial hazards that can occur across the life course and are known to have a detrimental impact on current and/or future health. These adversities include environmental *material* hazards such as poor nutrition, exposure to infections as a result of poor sanitation or inadequate access to drinking water, poor housing, unsafe road transport, poor neighbourhoods, and exposure to environmental toxins and teratogens (Abu-Saad and Fraser, 2010; Black et al., 2003; Black et al., 2008; Bolte, Tamburlini and Kohlhuber, 2010; Braubach and Fairburn, 2010; Grantham-McGregor et al., 2007; Hipp and Lakon, 2010; Kawachi and Berkman, 2003; Leventhal and Newman, 2010; Roux and Mair, 2010). They also include *psychosocial* hazards such as social exclusion, low status, low control, discrimination, abuse, victimisation, harsh and inconsistent parenting, witnessing domestic or community violence, and exposure to a range of other adverse 'life events' (Anda et al., 2006; Arseneault, Bowes and Shakoor, 2010; Bzostek and Beck, 2011; Carpenter and Stacks, 2009; Conger and Donnellan, 2007; Fowler et al., 2009; Gee et al., 2009; Gilbert et al., 2009; Glaser, 2008; Hoeve et al., 2009; Irish, Kobayashi and Delahanty, 2010; Jenkins, 2008; Jones, 2008; Krieger, 1999; Livingston and Boyd, 2010; Mays, Cochran and Barnes, 2007; Paradies, 2006; Rutter et al., 2009; Sandberg and Rutter, 2008; Turner, Finkelhor and Ormrod, 2006; Waldfogel, Craigie and Brooks-Gunn, 2010; Wegman and Stetler, 2009).

Risk of exposure to (and the severity of) specific environmental adversities will vary across cultures and time. So, for example, a child growing up in sub-Saharan Africa today may have a significant risk of exposure to some severe material hazards (e.g. severe under-nutrition, infectious disease, malaria) that may have a critical impact on their chances of survival and, if they survive, their cognitive, physical and emotional development (Black et al., 2003; Black et al., 2008; Grantham-McGregor et al., 2007). In contrast, for a child growing up in the UK or the USA risk of exposure to such severe material hazards will be very rare. However, risk of exposure to psychosocial hazards may be high and may play an important role in shaping their current and future well-being.

In all countries and at all times, however, it appears that risk of exposure to environmental adversities is unevenly distributed in populations. Rather, risk of exposure is typically patterned by socio- economic position (SEP). SEP refers to a person's position or standing in the social hierarchy, a position that is determined (in large part) by a process of social stratification involving key social institutions such as educational systems and the labour market (Graham, 2007). Membership of particular social groups (whether defined by wealth, gender, ethnicity, caste, religion, kinship ties, disability status, sexual orientation) may at particular times in particular cultures either privilege or act as barriers to accessing such social goods as education, employment, property and power. Lower SEP is also associated with higher risk of exposure to most (though not all) environmental adversities (Arseneault et al., 2010; Black et al., 2003; Bolte et al., 2010; Braubach and Fairburn, 2010; Carpenter and Stacks, 2009; Conger and Donnellan, 2007; Gilbert et al., 2009; Glaser, 2008; Grantham-McGregor et al., 2007; Hipp and Lakon, 2010; Jenkins, 2008; Jones, 2008; Kawachi and Berkman, 2003; Roux and Mair, 2010; Sandberg and Rutter, 2008; Van de Poel et al., 2008; Waldfogel et al., 2010).

Whilst an association between exposure to environmental adversities and poorer health has been repeatedly documented, recent research has significantly added to this knowledge in four areas. First, *life course approaches* to understanding health inequalities have highlighted the importance of the *cumulative exposure* to *multiple adversities* (including more mundane or everyday adversities) *across the life course* in directly and indirectly shaping health and well-being (Davey Smith, 2002; Graham, 2007). Indirect effects include the cascading effects that impact of exposure to adversity in early childhood may have on developmental health and through this on subsequent life experiences. For example, exposure to poverty in early childhood may impede a child's social and cognitive development, thereby reducing their 'readiness' to take advantage of developmental opportunities when starting school. Reduced 'school readiness' increases the risk of lower educational attainment. Low educational attainment has, in turn, been associated with downward social mobility and increased risk of unemployment or employment in precarious or insecure occupations, conditions that have been shown to be detrimental to health. Thus, whilst the cumulative effects of exposure to adversities across the life course are important in understanding health, exposure in early life, including prenatally, may be particularly important in also influencing a child's developmental health and consequently its risk of exposure to subsequent adversities in later life (Irwin, Siddiqi and Hertzman, 2007).

Second, research has begun to identify the complex social, psychological and biological pathways through which exposure to adversity may reduce health and well-being. Social pathways include the impact of poverty on parenting practices; associations partially mediated by the impact of poverty on parental stress and mental health, relationship quality and reduced financial opportunities for investment in activities that enhance child development (Conger and Donnellan, 2007). The limited research on psychological pathways has suggested that 'self-efficacy' may be partially determined by exposure to environmental adversities and consequently determine (in part) future life opportunities and responses to adversity (Matthews, Gallo and Taylor, 2010). Finally, it is clear that exposure to adversity can have a long-term impact on the development and functioning of biological systems in ways that increase the risk for poorer health: a process often referred to as 'biological embedding' or the pathways through which experience 'gets under the skin' (Hertzman and Boyce, 2010; McEwen and Gianaros, 2010; Miller, Chen and Parker, 2011; Shonkoff, 2010; Shonkoff, Boyce and McEwen, 2009). Attention, in particular, has focused on the notion of *allostatic load*, 'the wear-and-tear on the body and brain resulting from chronic dysregulation of physiological systems that are normally involved in adaptation to environmental challenge' (McEwen and Gianaros, 2010), specifically dysregulation of the hypothalamic–pituitary–adrenal (HPA) axis. The HPA axis responds to stressful circumstances by increasing the secretion of cortisol, a hormone that has metabolic effects on the brain and the immune, gastrointestinal, cardiovascular and other biological systems. Dysregulation of the HPA axis can lead to maladaptive wear and tear on these systems under chronically stressful conditions (Hertzman and Boyce, 2010; McEwen and Gianaros, 2010; Shonkoff, 2010; Shonkoff et al., 2009). Other models have focused on the impact of exposure to stress in early life on the long-term response tendencies of macrophages, cells that play a key role in initiating and maintaining inflammation (Miller et al., 2011).

Third, increasing attention has been paid over the last three decades to the differential vulnerability or resilience of people when exposed to adversity (Davydov et al., 2010; Jenkins, 2008; Luthar, 2003, 2006; Luthar and Brown, 2007; Luthar, Sawyer and Brown, 2006; Masten, 2001; Mohaupt, 2009; Rutter, 1979, 1985; Schoon, 2006; Ungar, 2008; Werner and Smith, 1992). This body of research has highlighted the extent to which understanding resilience requires looking beyond the characteristics of individuals. Factors promoting resilience include not only individual characteristics of the child (e.g. problem-solving skills, intelligence, temperament), but also the characteristics of the context in which children live including the characteristics of families, the child's relationship within its family, the characteristics of communities and the child's relationship with those communities.

Finally, the recent focus on understanding and quantifying the causal role of these 'social determinants' of health has highlighted the social significance of these processes for understanding and addressing the stark inequalities in the distribution of health that occur across and within populations (The Marmot Review, 2010; World Health Organization, 2008, 2013; World Health Organization Regional Office for Europe, 2010b). That is not to say that the association between increased rates of exposure to adversities and poorer health is a simple one-way process. As suggested above, poorer developmental health in childhood can constrain upward social mobility, leading in later life to lower SEP with an associated increased risk of exposure to additional adversities. To the extent to which upward social mobility may be influenced by characteristics that have some hereditable genetic component (e.g. general intelligence, though this is a contested issue) *and* that these characteristics are related to health (Batty, Deary and Gottfredson, 2007; Batty et al., 2006; Batty et al., 2009; Calvin et al., 2011), a degree of the association between increased rates of exposure to adversities and poorer health may be attributable to the consequences of genetics. What has become clear, however, is that the main reason for the association between increased rates of exposure to adversities and poorer health is that exposure to adversities damages health and that differential rates of exposure to adversities are very clearly unnecessary, avoidable, unfair and unjust.

Taken together, this increasingly mature body of knowledge makes a compelling case that in trying to account for the poorer health or well-being of a particular group of people within any population at any period of time, it would be wise to examine the potential role played by differential exposure to common 'social determinants' of health. For example, the preamble to the recent Rio Political Declaration on Social Determinants of Health, which was adopted by UN Member States in October 2011, summarises the importance of this body of knowledge thus:

> Health inequities arise from the societal conditions in which people are born, grow, live, work and age, referred to as social determinants of health. These include early years' experiences, education, economic status, employment and decent work, housing and environment, and effective systems of preventing and treating ill health. We are convinced that action on these determinants, both for vulnerable groups and the entire population, is essential to create inclusive, equitable, economically productive and healthy societies.[2]

In Chapter 4 we will apply this approach to understanding the poorer health of people with intellectual disabilities.

---

[2] www.who.int/sdhconference/declaration/en.

The health of people with intellectual disabilities

Over the last decade numerous review papers, reports and books have summarised what is known about the (generally poorer) health of people with intellectual disabilities (Elliott, Hatton and Emerson, 2003; Emerson et al., 2012a; Fisher, 2004; Graham, 2005; Haveman et al., 2010; Heslop et al., 2013; Krahn and Fox, in press; Krahn, Hammond and Turner, 2006; NHS Health Scotland, 2004; Nocon, 2006; O'Hara, McCarthy and Bouras, 2010b; Oeseburg et al., 2011; Ouellette-Kuntz, 2005; Perry et al., 2011; Prasher and Janicki, 2003; Scheepers et al., 2005; Shogren et al., 2006; Sutherland, Couch and Iacono, 2002; US Department of Health and Human Services, 2002b; Van Schrojenstein Lantman-de Valk, 2005; Van Schrojenstein Lantman-de Valk and Walsh, 2008). Our aim in this chapter is to summarise what the available research literature tells us about the health status and needs of children and adults with intellectual disabilities. Given the availability of previous reviews (see above), we will focus on the 'big picture' and on more recent evidence as it relates to broad indicators of health (e.g. overall mortality, self-rated health) and specific health conditions and impairments. Before doing that, however, we need to understand the strengths and limitations of the existing evidence base and the implications that these have for our understanding of the health inequalities faced by people with intellectual disabilities.

Evaluating the evidence base

The sheer volume of scientific papers, reports, book chapters and books that have been written about different aspects of the health of people with intellectual disabilities can give the impression that a good robust evidence base exists that can inform our understanding and thereby provide a sturdy foundation for action. Unfortunately, that is not quite the case. It is important to keep two questions in mind when judging the robustness of the existing evidence: Which people with intellectual disabilities participated in the research? How was health measured?

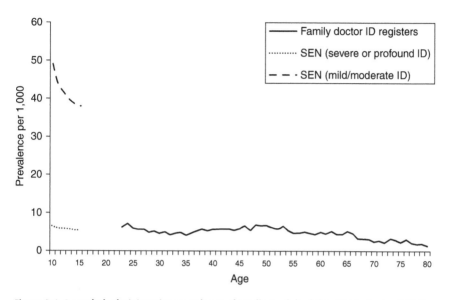

Figure 3.1 Recorded administrative prevalence of intellectual disability (ID) in England 2010 (from Emerson and Glover, 2012) (SEN, special educational needs)

Which people with intellectual disabilities participate in research?

A central aim of this book is to apply a public health (and health inequalities) lens to understanding and ameliorating the health inequalities experienced by people with intellectual disabilities. As a result, we are interested in understanding the health (and the determinants of health) of *all* people with intellectual disabilities that live in a particular society or locality. To do this we need information on health (and its determinants) that is representative of the population with which we are concerned (e.g. people with intellectual disabilities living in England, people with intellectual disabilities living in Northern Sydney).

Unfortunately, very few studies provide this kind of information. This is especially the case for studies that examine the health of adults with intellectual disability. This problem arises because the vast majority of research studies involving people with intellectual disabilities draw their participants from *administrative samples* of people with intellectual disabilities who are known to or are using specialised intellectual disability services (Centers for Disease Control and Prevention (CDC) and National Center on Birth Defects and Developmental Disabilities (NCBDDD) Health Surveillance Work Group, 2009; Krahn and Fox, in press; Krahn et al., 2010). This would not be problematic if all people with intellectual disabilities were known to or were using specialised intellectual disability services (or if this group of users was representative of the wider population of non-users). This is simply not the case.

The problem can be illustrated by charting the known *administrative prevalence* (i.e. prevalence based on administrative samples) of intellectual disability across different ages and comparing this with what is known from the epidemiological research we discussed in Chapter 1 about the 'true' prevalence of intellectual disability. Figure 3.1 (taken from Emerson and Glover, 2012) does this for people with intellectual disabilities in England using data available for 2010/11. It shows estimates of the age-specific administrative prevalence of intellectual disability for single-year age groups. For children, data from the English Department for Education's National Pupil Database was used. This includes information on children attending maintained (state-funded) schools and non-maintained (non-profit-making independent) special schools (information that covers approximately 98% of all English children). For adults, we used information collected by the English NHS Information Centre for Health and Social Care on the total number of adults (aged 18+) whom general practitioners (GPs) had identified as having intellectual disabilities. This total figure was then combined with data extracted from eight local areas to estimate the likely age profile of this group. The base for the prevalence estimates was population estimates from the UK's Office for National Statistics.

As can be seen, there is an obvious 'transition cliff' in Figure 3.1, with the administrative prevalence dropping precipitously within a couple of years of age from around 40–50 per 1000 to 6–7 per 1000. Similar abrupt declines in age-specific administrative prevalence rates have also been reported in the USA (Campbell and Fedeyko, 2001; Kiely, 1987; National Center on Birth Defects and Developmental Disabilities, 2010).

The marked discrepancy between the administrative prevalence of intellectual disability in adult services and estimates of the 'true' prevalence of learning disability has been commented on previously (Emerson and Hatton, 2008a; Emerson et al., 2011e; Whitaker, 2004). This discrepancy almost certainly reflects the very low rates of use of specialised intellectual disability services amongst adults with less-severe intellectual disability (whether by choice or exclusion). (Note the similarity between the administrative prevalence of severe or profound intellectual disability in childhood and of intellectual disability in adulthood.) Invisible in administrative statistics, this group of adults with predominantly mild intellectual disability has been referred to as the 'hidden majority' of adults with intellectual disabilities (Edgerton, 2001; Tymchuk, Lakin and Luckasson, 2001).

There are two points here that are important. First, virtually all that we know about the health of adults with intellectual disabilities is based on studies of the 'visible minority' of adults with (predominantly severe or profound) intellectual disabilities, who use specialised intellectual disability services. Whilst very little is known about the health of the 'hidden majority', the available evidence suggests that, when compared with their non-disabled peers, they are more likely to: have poorer health; be exposed to social conditions detrimental to positive health; and to engage in more risky health behaviours (Campbell and Fedeyko, 2001; Emerson, 2011; Snell and Luckasson, 2009; Tymchuk, Lakin and Luckasson, 2001). Second, given that the majority of people with more severe intellectual disabilities are likely to be known to or using specialised intellectual disability services, using administrative samples is probably a quite reasonable strategy for understanding their health. However, it is likely to be a deeply flawed strategy for understanding the health of the *majority* of adults with intellectual disabilities (who will have mild intellectual disability). This is particularly the case given that people with less severe intellectual disabilities are likely to be known by or using such services precisely because they have significant additional healthcare needs.

This is an important issue as the health needs of the 'hidden majority' may be quite different from the health needs of the 'visible minority'. For example, the two leading global risks for mortality in the world are high blood pressure (responsible for 13% of deaths globally) and tobacco use (responsible for 9% of deaths globally) (World Health Organization, 2009). Numerous studies have reported low rates of tobacco use amongst people with intellectual disabilities (Beange, McElduff and Baker, 1995; Fidler, Michell and Charlton, 1992; Glover, Emerson, and Eccles, 2012a; Rimmer, Braddock and Marks, 1995; Robertson et al., 2000b; Wee et al., in press). But how representative is this evidence, based as it is on administrative samples, of people with intellectual disabilities more generally? It is possibly highly misleading given the evidence that adolescents (especially boys) with mild intellectual disabilities are more likely to smoke than their peers (Emerson and Turnbull, 2005; Emerson et al., 2011a) and that rates of smoking are higher amongst adults with mild intellectual disability who do not use services when compared with those who do (Emerson, 2011).

How is health measured?

Health is a broad concept, and research on health covers a multitude of methods and techniques including: laboratory analysis of physical specimens (e.g. Hsu et al., 2012b); the analysis of large-scale health surveys (e.g. Schieve et al., 2012) and administrative records (e.g. Jensen and Davis, 2013); medical examination (e.g. Wee et al., in press); and self- and carer reports of health (e.g. Turk et al., 2012). For some of these approaches (e.g. laboratory analysis of physical specimens) the challenges associated with undertaking research are not particularly different when the participants are people with intellectual disabilities. For other methods, undertaking research with a focus on intellectual disability involves some particular challenges that we briefly discuss in the following sections.

Large-scale Health Surveys

Research based on the analysis of existing large-scale health surveys and longitudinal studies (commonly termed secondary analysis) is commonplace in public health. Secondary analysis has been used in our field to investigate such issues as factors associated with the emotional and behavioural development of young children with intellectual disabilities (Emerson, 2012c; Emerson and Einfeld, 2010; Emerson, Einfeld and Stancliffe, 2011b; Totsika and Hastings, 2012) and the prevalence of intellectual disabilities (Larson, Lakin and Anderson, 2003; Larson et al., 2001b). There are, however, two particular challenges involved in secondary analysis when applied to the study of intellectual disabilities: (1) identifying people with intellectual disabilities who may have participated in the survey; and (2) the limitations of general population sampling strategies.

It is rare indeed for major surveys to be designed with the explicit intention of identifying whether participants have an intellectual disability. As a result, the first task when examining a potential data source is to determine whether it will be possible to design a method that can credibly identify participants who may have an intellectual disability. Whilst this is commonly possible in birth cohort and child development surveys, it has proved much more problematic for surveys of adult populations. There are three general strategies for identifying survey participants who may have intellectual disability: (1) data linkage to administrative data sets; (2) classification based on cognitive and/or psychological testing; and (3) self- or informant reports.

Whilst rare at present, there is a growing trend to link (with consent) survey data to administrative data held by government departments. In the UK, for example, two national surveys (the Longitudinal Study of Young People in England, and child data from Understanding Society) have been linked to information held by the English Department for Education on whether the child has been identified through educational systems as having intellectual disability (for an example of how this can be used, see Emerson and Halpin, 2013).

Children's cognitive development is a key outcome of interest in most large-scale birth cohort and child development studies. As a result, these studies typically undertake brief cognitive testing of child participants at different stages of their lives. As these are population-based studies, it therefore becomes a relatively simple task to use these test scores to identify children with intellectual disability on the basis of them scoring two standard deviations below the weighted sample mean on these tests or having not been tested due to their cognitive impairments (e.g. Emerson et al., 2010). Whilst such an approach is sufficiently robust to identify children with intellectual disability according to ICD-10 criteria, it is insufficient to identify children with intellectual disability by DSM-IV or AAIDD criteria (Einfeld and Emerson, 2008).

Child-focused surveys that do not involve either data linkage or cognitive testing will often collect parental reports of the presence of child impairments or disabilities or receipt of professional diagnosis associated with intellectual disabilities. Little is currently known about the validity of parental responses to these types of questions and the extent to which the accuracy of informant reports may be moderated by potentially important contextual factors (Emerson, Felce and Stancliffe, in press).

The identification of adults with intellectual disability in large-scale surveys is much more problematic, though not impossible (see, for example, Larson et al., 2001b). An increasing number of surveys collect information on whether the adult respondent has a disability and, if so, the type(s) of impairments associated with their disability. The list of impairments from which the participant can select often contains an item such as 'difficulty learning or understanding'. It is sometimes possible to combine responses to this item with other information contained within the survey (e.g. very low educational attainment, difficulties with literacy and numeracy) to operationally identify a sub-group of adults who may have intellectual disability. However, a recent review of 123 European health surveys reported that only 7 contained information that could potentially be used to identify people with intellectual disabilities (Linehan et al., 2009).

The important issue with regard to sampling is that most population-based surveys use 'general households' as the primary sampling unit. Whilst this ensures coverage of the vast majority of the population, it excludes people who are either homeless or living in some form of institutional arrangement. Whilst there is no reliable information on the extent of homelessness amongst people with intellectual disabilities, it is clear that a significant proportion of adults with intellectual disabilities who are known to services live in supported accommodation arrangements, some of which are likely to be excluded from samples of 'general households'.

A final barrier to identifying participants with intellectual disabilities is that they may have been excluded from the sample due to their perceived inability to either give consent to or to participate effectively in the survey. It is extremely rare for large-scale population-based surveys to incorporate 'reasonable accommodations' to the survey process (e.g. simplifying and rephrasing questions, use of visual aids) that would facilitate the participation of people with intellectual disabilities (Emerson et al., 2005).

Use of administrative records

Research based on the analysis of administrative data is also commonplace in public health research. It has been used in our field to investigate such issues as variation in the prevalence of intellectual and developmental disabilities (Chapman, Scott and Stanton-Chapman, 2008; Emerson, 2012a; Leonard et al., 2003, 2005, 2008), the health and healthcare received by people with intellectual disabilities (Balogh, Hunter and Ouellette-Kuntz, 2005; Balogh et al., 2010; Glover and Evison, 2013; Thomas et al., 2011), and mortality (Glover and Ayub, 2010).

However, the identification of people with intellectual disabilities in administrative data sets can also be problematic (Lin et al., 2013; Westerinen et al., 2007). Data sets maintained by specialised intellectual disability services face all the problems of representativeness that we discussed above. However, there are numerous generic administrative systems (e.g. of hospital admissions, death certification, welfare payments) within which it may be possible to identify people with intellectual disabilities.

The validity of the data extracted from these systems will depend crucially on the accuracy of the coding system employed to identify individuals with intellectual disabilities, or with conditions associated with intellectual or developmental disabilities (e.g. Down's syndrome) (Glover and Emerson, 2012a). As we have seen (Figure 3.1), issues of coding accuracy are particularly problematic in identifying people with less severe intellectual disability in generic administrative data sets (i.e. those not collected by intellectual disability agencies).

However, the under-identification of people with intellectual disabilities (including people with severe intellectual disabilities) in generic health-related data systems appears to be widespread. For example, in a recent study based on death certification in the UK, just 0.04% of certificates stated that the person had an intellectual disability (compared with an approximate prevalence of severe intellectual disability of 0.35%). In this instance, however, it was possible to increase the capture rate by also including people identified as having conditions or syndromes typically associated with intellectual disability (e.g. Down's syndrome, which was identified on 0.09% of certificates). Similarly, the presence of intellectual disability is supposed to be recorded (using ICD-10 codes) for all hospital episodes in England. However, only 0.05% of hospital episodes use the appropriate ICD-10 codes (F70–F799), although the code 'F819' ('Developmental disorder of scholastic skills, unspecified') is used much more frequently (0.23% of episodes), apparently as an alternative given the pejorative terminology used in ICD-10 to describe intellectual disability ('mental retardation') (Glover and Emerson, 2012a). Tracking individuals over time in such systems can increase the identification rate (e.g. by identifying people who have ever been identified as having intellectual disability). However, the use of different methods to identify people with intellectual disabilities in administrative data sets may produce different results, not only in terms of overall prevalence, but also in terms of the health characteristics of the population identified. In a recent study undertaken in Canada, for example, the use of a more stringent approach to identifying people with intellectual disabilities from administrative data identified much higher rates of mental health problems amongst people with intellectual disabilities than two less stringent approaches (Lin et al., 2013).

When interpreting the results of research based on administrative data sets, careful consideration needs to be given to the types of biases that may be operating in identifying people with intellectual or developmental disabilities. For example, GPs in England are identifying increasing numbers of adults as having intellectual disability (Emerson et al., 2013). Does this reflect a true increase in the number of adults with intellectual disability in England or is this rise driven by other factors (e.g. the introduction of financial incentives to GPs to provide annual health checks for adults with intellectual disability)? Does the marked increase in the recorded prevalence of autism in many countries reflect a real rise in prevalence, an increase in the accuracy of identification (assuming a history of under-identification), a broadening of the concept of autism or the over-diagnosis of autism, driven in some areas by the diagnosis giving access to additional resources or services (Elsabbagh et al., 2012; Newschaffer et al., 2007)?

Table 3.1 Percentage of survey participants with intellectual disability (ID) who were considered to reliably self-report on their general health status (data extracted from Emerson et al., 2005)

	In contact with ID services	Not in contact with ID services
Living in private household alone or with partner	85	86
Living in private household with relatives	28	59
Living in supported accommodation	43	n/a

Self-report and proxy responding

An individual's capacity to monitor, reflect on and report on aspects of their health plays a crucial role in many approaches to health measurement. Within international classificatory systems many diagnoses (especially of mental health disorders) require information through self-report. Some aspects of health (e.g. pain) are only accessible through self-report. Most health measurement scales and questionnaires are dependent on self-report (McDowell, 2006). This gives rise to some challenges and dilemmas in assessing the health of people with intellectual disabilities (Fujiura, 2012), especially if we wish to make comparisons between the health of people with intellectual disabilities and their non-disabled peers. We need to keep four questions in mind when evaluating how trustworthy our evidence base is when it uses self-report measures:

1. To what extent can people with intellectual disabilities use self-report measures that have been developed for the general population?
2. What impact does making 'reasonable adjustments' (e.g. simplified wording) to standard self-report measures or diagnostic systems to maximise the participation of people with intellectual disabilities have on the validity of the information collected?
3. If a person cannot self-report, does proxy reporting (e.g. carer report) represent a valid alternative?
4. If a person cannot self-report, do we need to change diagnostic criteria?

Much has been written about the difficulties experienced by some people with intellectual disabilities in self-reporting on aspects of their experience, including their health, and of the specific risks for acquiescent responding (agreeing with the question) and response bias (e.g. using just the extreme points of response scales) (e.g. Finlay and Lyons, 2001; Fujiura, 2012; Hartley and MacLean, 2006; Prosser and Bromley, 2012). But how common are these difficulties? The answer (predictably) is that it depends on which group of people with intellectual disabilities we are concerned with: the visible minority of people with more severe intellectual disability or the hidden majority of people with less severe intellectual disability. To illustrate this, Table 3.1 presents information on the percentage of survey participants with intellectual disability who were considered to reliably self-report on their general health status (data extracted from Emerson et al., 2005).

As can be seen, whilst a significant majority of people with intellectual disabilities not in contact with intellectual disability services were able to self-report on their general health status, only a minority of those in contact with intellectual disability services were able to do so (apart from the 5% of those in contact with intellectual disability services who were living independently). Similarly high rates of ability to self-report have been observed in population-based samples of adolescents with intellectual disability (Emerson, 2005b).

One response to the low rates of self-reporting amongst people with more severe intellectual disability has been to make 'reasonable adjustments' (e.g. simplified wording, use of pictorial cues) to self-report measures to maximise the participation of people with intellectual disabilities (e.g. Finlay and Lyons, 2001; Fujiura, 2012; Hartley and MacLean, 2006; Hatton and Taylor, 2013; Prosser and Bromley, 2012). Whilst such adjustments may be successful in increasing response rates, it is unclear how comparable the resulting information may be with that produced by the unaltered standardised scale.

An enduring concern with assessing the health and well-being of people with intellectual disabilities is the validity and acceptability of collecting information from proxy respondents (typically paid or unpaid carers) when the person themselves does not have the capacity to answer. The research that has been undertaken in this area has primarily focused on two areas: (1) evaluating the degree of agreement between people with intellectual disabilities and carers; and (2) evaluating the degree of agreement between carer report and professional evaluation of health status.

For obvious reasons it is only possible to evaluate the degree of agreement between people with intellectual disabilities and carers if both parties are capable of self-reporting and, as Roger Stancliffe has commented, 'it remains an open question as to whether findings of agreement between proxies and self-reports from verbal individuals can be generalized to non-verbal people with more profound intellectual disability who cannot respond for themselves' (Stancliffe, 2000). Nevertheless, this body of research has highlighted the variable and at times very poor degree of agreement between people with intellectual disabilities and carers, especially for reporting internal states and feelings (Cummins, 2002; Perry, 2004; Stancliffe, 2000). To give a recent example, Vicky Turk and colleagues compared self-report and carers' responses to a simple health checklist for 59 adults with intellectual disabilities (Turk et al., 2012). They reported good agreement for two items (epilepsy and asthma), moderate agreement for five items (ear problems, eye problems, weight problems, skin problems and allergies) and poor agreement for the remaining nine items (including depression, anxiety, headache/migraine and dental problems). There is also a small body of evidence that suggests that carers of people with intellectual disabilities may perceive the person they care for to be healthier than suggested by the results of medical examinations (Beange et al., 1995; Wilson and Haire, 1990). Clearly, proxy responses are imperfect substitutes for self-report and should be used with considerable caution.

If the use of proxy responses is problematic, then the identification of some health conditions (particularly mental health disorders) becomes particularly problematic amongst people with severe intellectual disabilities who may not be able to communicate their thoughts, feelings and internal states. As such, it is unclear how applicable diagnostic systems developed to classify mental health problems are to people with intellectual disability (Cooper, 2004; Cooper et al., 2007a, 2007b; Dagnan, 2007; Sturmey, 2007). For example, can a person with no symbolic language experience auditory hallucinations, or have the cognitive skills necessary to conceptualise and plan a suicide attempt? Whilst modified diagnostic criteria have been produced for people with mild learning disabilities (World Health Organization, 1996) and people with moderate to severe learning disabilities (Royal College of Psychiatrists, 2001), such modifications have been the subject of debate, being based on informal expert consensus methods with limited validity (Cooper, 2003; Einfeld and Tonge, 1999).

In the following sections we will summarise what the available research literature tells us about the health status and needs of children and adults with intellectual disabilities. We will start with evidence that relates to general indicators of health status (mortality and self-reported general health) before moving on to specific health conditions and impairments.

General indicators of health

Mortality

People with intellectual disabilities have a shorter life expectancy (DeSalvo et al., 2006) and increased age-specific mortality rates *across all ages* when compared with the general population (Bittles et al., 2002; Glover and Ayub, 2010; Hollins et al., 1998; McGuigan, Hollins and Attard, 1995). For some groups of people with intellectual disabilities, life expectancy has shown marked increases over the past few decades (Baird and Sadovnick, 1988). For example, the life expectancy of people with Down's syndrome increased from 9 years in 1929 to 49 in 1997 (Yang, Rasmussen and Friedman, 2002). In high-income countries, recent estimates indicate that the mean age of death for people with Down's syndrome is greater than 50 years (Coppus et al., 2008). There is some evidence from Finland to suggest that the life expectancy of people with mild intellectual disabilities is approaching that of the general population (Patja et al., 2000). However, recent data from England indicate that the median age of death of people with mild intellectual disabilities remains considerably younger than that of the general population (for men 71 vs 78 years; for women 65 vs 83 years) (Heslop et al., 2013). All-cause mortality rates amongst people with moderate to severe

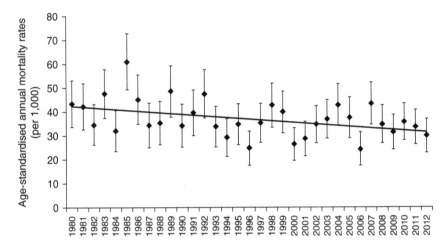

Figure 3.2 Age-standardised annual mortality rates (with 95% confidence intervals and best fit linear projection) for people with intellectual disabilities in Sheffield, England, 1980–2012

intellectual disabilities remain three times higher than in the general population, with mortality being particularly high for people with more severe disabilities, young adults, women, people with epilepsy, and people with Down's syndrome and other genetic causes of intellectual disability (Bittles et al., 2002; Patja et al., 2000; Tyrer and McGrother, 2009).

Reductions over time in mortality rates for people with intellectual disabilities are illustrated in Figure 3.2. This figure uses annual mortality data extracted from the Sheffield Case Register from 1980 to 2012. The mortality rates have been standardised to a 'standard European population' to take account of changes in the age profile of people with intellectual disabilities over this period of time (London Health Observatory, undated). Whilst there is marked year-on-year variability due to the relatively small numbers of people with learning disabilities (just over 100 deaths per year in a population of 7000–10,000 people with intellectual disabilities), there is a significant downward linear trend in mortality. This is equivalent to a 1.2% year-on-year reduction in mortality rates. However, over the same period annual age-standardised mortality rates in the general population in England and Wales declined by 2.2% for men and 1.7% for women (Office for National Statistics, 2012). As such, the *relative inequality* in mortality rates showed a modest increase over this period.

One key issue (and one to which we will return) is the extent to which the higher mortality rates amongst people with intellectual disabilities reflect an excess of preventable or premature deaths. For example, potentially preventable causes of death that are relatively common and affect most groups of people with intellectual disabilities include aspiration pneumonia and other respiratory diseases, seizures and cardiovascular disease (Glover and Ayub, 2010; Patja, Mölsä and Iivanainen,

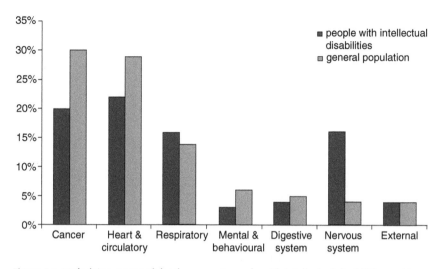

Figure 3.3 Underlying causes of death amongst people with intellectual disabilities and in the general population (data taken from Heslop et al., 2013)

2001). A recent investigation of the causes and circumstances of 244 deaths of people with intellectual disabilities in England concluded that: (1) 42% were premature in that specific adverse events were identified in the pathway leading to death that if prevented would probably have allowed the person to live for at least another year; and (2) 28% were 'amenable' in that in light of current knowledge, all or most deaths from that cause could have been avoided through the provision of good-quality healthcare (Heslop et al., 2013). Amongst a subset of 58 of these deaths matched with 58 deaths from the same causes at the same age and in the same locality amongst people without intellectual disabilities, the deaths of people with intellectual disabilities were more likely to be premature (52% vs 43%) and amenable (38% vs 9%) (Heslop et al., 2013).

Figure 3.3 presents information on the underlying causes of death amongst this cohort of people with intellectual disabilities and amongst deaths in the general population of England and Wales for the same time period.

As can be seen, people with intellectual disabilities were proportionately less likely to die from cancer and heart and circulatory disorders (the two leading underlying causes of death in England and Wales in 2011) than people in the general population. They were marginally more likely to die from respiratory disorders and much more likely to die from disorders of the nervous system (most commonly deaths associated with epilepsy or cerebral palsy). Similar patterns in relation to cause of death (and differences between people with and without intellectual disabilities) have been reported from mortality reviews undertaken in Massachusetts (Lauer, 2010, 2012) and Connecticut (Department of Developmental Services, 2011, 2012).

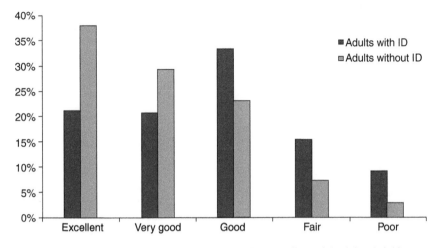

Figure 3.4 Self-rated health of US adults with and without intellectual disability (ID) (data taken from Larson et al., 2001a)

General health status

Ratings of general health status are commonly used as indicators of the health of populations. They are easy to collect and predict current and future morbidity and future mortality (DeSalvo et al., 2006; Fujiura, 2012; Idler and Benyamini, 1997, 1999; Jylha, 2009). Numerous health surveys ask adult respondents to rate their overall health status and parental informants to rate the overall health status of their children.

The risk of children being reported by their main carers (usually their mothers) to have fair/poor general health is 2.5–4.5 times greater for children with intellectual disabilities when compared with their non-disabled peers (Emerson and Hatton, 2007a, 2007c). One in seven adults with predominantly mild intellectual disabilities in England rates their general health as not good (Emerson and Hatton, 2008c). To our knowledge, only two large-scale population-based studies have compared the self-rated health of adults with intellectual disabilities with their non-disabled peers (Department of Health, 2011; Larson et al., 2001a). Sheryl Larson and colleagues used data collected in the disability supplements to the US National Health Interview Survey (NHIS) to identify respondents with predominantly mild intellectual disability and to compare their health status and service use with their non-disabled peers (Larson et al., 2001b, 2003). Figure 3.4 summarises information from their Data Brief (Larson et al., 2001a) on the self-reported health of American adults with and without intellectual disability.

As can be seen, adults with intellectual disability were markedly more likely to rate their health as fair or poor (24%) than their peers without intellectual disability (10%). Similar results were obtained in a state-wide study of the health of adults with intellectual disability in the Australian state of Victoria (Department of Health, 2011). Whilst there are considerable difficulties in using self-report measures, especially amongst people with more severe intellectual disability (Fujiura, 2012), these figures are consistent with the evidence we have reviewed above on mortality and the evidence we will review below on the prevalence of specific health conditions and impairments.

Specific health conditions and impairments

In the following sections we provide an overview of evidence that relates to the prevalence of specific health conditions and impairments amongst people with intellectual disabilities. We have used the WHO's International Classification of Functioning, Disability and Health (ICF) to structure this section (World Health Organization, 2001). We will begin by examining some examples of the small number of studies that have attempted to determine the prevalence of a wide range of health conditions and impairments in people with and without intellectual disabilities using either population-based surveys or by extracting information from primary healthcare data systems.

Table 3.2 summarises the results of two population-based surveys that address the health of children with and without intellectual disability: a UK study that used parental report on the health of 7-year-old children (465 with intellectual disability, 10,572 without intellectual disability) collected in the Millennium Cohort Study (Emerson et al., 2011a); and a US study that used parental report on the health of 3–17-year-old children (238 with intellectual disability but not autism, 35,775 without disability) collected in the 2006–10 National Health Interview Surveys (Schieve et al., 2012).

What is striking about the data presented in this table is that, despite the different locations, age ranges and methods used, both studies report poorer health status for children with intellectual disability when compared with their peers across a very wide range of specific health conditions and, for the UK study, health risks. On no indicator of health status or health risk did children with intellectual disability have significantly better health than their non-disabled peers. On 22 of the 28 measures (79%) across the two studies, children with intellectual disability had significantly poorer health than their non-disabled peers.

Table 3.3 summarises the results of four population-based surveys that address the health of adults with and without intellectual disability. First, a seminal study undertaken by Helen Beange and colleagues, who examined the health of a random sample of 202 Australian adults with intellectual disability aged 20–50 (Beange et al., 1995). Second, a state-wide telephone survey (using proxy respondents) of the health of 897 adults with intellectual disability in the state of Victoria, Australia (Department of Health, 2011) using questions and methods similar to other state health surveys. Finally, two studies, one undertaken in the UK, the other in the Netherlands, both using information from primary healthcare services to compare

Table 3.2 Health of children with intellectual disabilities (ID; %), and odds ratio (OR)

Study	UK: Emerson et al. (2011a)			US: Schieve et al. (2012)		
	ID	No ID	OR	ID	No ID	OR
Child health rated by parent as 'fair' or 'poor'	10	2	4.7*			
Health Conditions and Impairments						
Eyesight problems	28	17	2.0*			
Hearing problems	21	13	1.8*			
≥3 ear infections in previous year				10	4	3.3*
Epilepsy	4	1	3.0*	15	1	46.7*
Frequent severe headache/migraine				13	5	2.9*
Head/chest cold in previous 2 weeks				25	15	2.3*
Wheezing	35	27	1.4*			
Asthma	19	16	1.2	25	14	1.7*
Eczema	36	37	1.0	13	10	1.5
Hay fever	15	16	1.0			
Respiratory allergy				15	11	1.4
Digestive allergy				4	4	0.9
Frequent diarrhoea/colitis (previous year)				4	1	5.3*
Stomach/intestinal illness with vomiting or diarrhoea (previous 2 weeks)				12	5	2.9*
Conduct difficulties	23	9	3.3*			
Emotional difficulties	18	6	3.3*			
Hyperactivity	41	11	5.4*			

Peer problems	25	7	4.5*
≥3 of the above health problems	52	28	2.7*
Health Risks			
≥2 accidents requiring medical attention	9	4	2.2*
Obese	9	5	1.7*
Never does sport/exercise	56	25	3.8*
Lived in materially poor home at more than one point in time	44	20	3.3*
Bullied more than 'once or twice' at school	14	6	2.5*

Note: * difference statistically significant at $p < 0.05$

Table 3.3: Health of adults with intellectual disabilities (ID; %)

Study	Australia: Beange et al. (1995)		Australia: Department of Health (2011)		UK: Samele et al. (2006)		Netherlands: Straetmans et al. (2007)	
	ID (n = 202)	No ID (n = 807)	ID (n = 897)	No ID (n = 34,169)	ID (n = 753)	No ID (n = 149,428)	ID (n = 868)	No ID (n = 4305)
Health Conditions/ Impairments								
Cardiovascular disease	24	–	6	8				
Ischaemic heart disease					1	4		
Stroke			2	3	1	2		
Diabetes mellitus			9	6	2	3	11	6
Chronic obstructive pulmonary disease					20	16		
Upper respiratory tract infection							11	6
Migrane/headaches								
Epilepsy	29	1					17	<1
Acne	4	1						
Eczema							9	5
Dermatomycosis							12	6
Other infection of skin/ subcutis/erysipelas							7	1
Gastrointestinal disorders	17	–						
Constipation							5	<1

Food allergies						
Blindness	4	<1				
Deafness	25	2				
Excess ear wax					10	3
Health Risks						
Obesity	21	8	27	17	28	20
Hypertension	10	6			8	11
No exercise	74	58	78	40		
Smoking	6	47	6	19		
Drinking alcohol	25	87	34	82		
Health Screening						
Mamography (age ≥50)			55	76	35	40
Cervical screening			15	71	1	2
Total cholesterol					11	27
Urine analysis					24	30
Smoking status					15	25
Body mass index (BMI)					39	54
Systolic blood pressure			85	80	48	68
Diastolic blood pressure					47	67
Health Interventions						
Flu vaccination					25	22
Tetanus vaccination					33	36
Dietary advice					20	32

the recorded prevalence of particular health conditions and impairments, health risks and health interventions amongst relatively large samples of adults with and without intellectual disability (Samele et al., 2006; Straetmans et al., 2007). The UK study electronically extracted data from 22 GP practices across three English Primary Care Trusts and one Welsh Local Health Board (Samele et al., 2006). The Netherlands study used data collected in the Second Dutch National Survey of General Practice in 2001. This included information about consultations in 104 general practices covering 400,000 registered patients (Straetmans et al., 2007).

Again, what is striking about the data presented in this table is that all four studies report poorer health status for adults with intellectual disability when compared with their peers across a very wide range of specific health conditions and health risks and, for the UK study, lower rates of uptake of health screening interventions. We will return to this issue in the next chapter.

Mental functions

Mental health and challenging behaviour

The mental, emotional and behavioural health of people with intellectual disabilities is one of the most researched topics in the field of intellectual disability (Bouras and Holt, 2007; Dagnan and Lindsay, 2012; Emerson and Einfeld, 2011; Oeseburg et al., 2011; Ruedrich, 2010; Taylor et al., 2013). Despite this, there is surprisingly little robust information on the prevalence of mental health disorders amongst people (especially adults) with intellectual disabilities, and the extent to which they may be at greater (or lesser) risk than their non-disabled peers (Kerker et al., 2004).

There is growing evidence from a number of relatively well-constructed population-based studies that children with intellectual disabilities are more likely to have mental health and behavioural difficulties than their peers (Einfeld, Ellis and Emerson, 2011; Emerson and Einfeld, 2010; Emerson, Einfeld and Stancliffe, 2010; Emerson et al., 2011b). UK studies, for example, suggest that at any point in time 36% of children with intellectual disabilities have a diagnosable mental health disorder (using ICD-10 or DSM-V criteria), compared with just 8% of children without intellectual disabilities (Emerson, 2003; Emerson and Hatton, 2007b). As a result, children with intellectual disabilities account for 14% of all UK children with a diagnosable mental health disorder. It is important to note that this increased risk occurred across the range of mental health disorders, rather than being specific to particular types of disorder (Emerson and Hatton, 2007b).

There is also growing evidence that the prevalence of psychiatric disorders is significantly higher amongst adults who are identified by their GPs as having intellectual disability, when compared with general population prevalence rates, although to what extent depends on which diagnostic methods are used (Cooper et al., 2007a, 2007b; Department of Health, 2011; Glover et al., 2012a; Singleton et al., 2001). The problem here, however, is that GPs only identify a small proportion of those adults with mild intellectual disability who live in the community (Emerson and Glover, 2012). If GP identification of people with mild intellectual disability is more likely if the person also has mental health problems (not an unreasonable assumption), this would lead to an over-estimation of the prevalence of mental health problems amongst adults with intellectual disability. There are, however, good grounds for concluding on the bases of these studies that people with more severe intellectual disability (who are likely to be more reliably identified as such by their GPs) do have a higher risk of mental health problems.

There are also good grounds for assuming that people with less severe intellectual disability (including the 'hidden majority' of adults with mild intellectual disability) are likely to have a higher risk of mental health problems. First, several of the prevalence studies of child mental health referred to above are essentially studies of the mental health of children with mild intellectual disability. It is a little implausible to assume that their increased risk of mental health difficulties should vanish on reaching adulthood. Second, the small numbers of studies that have investigated the well-being of community-based samples of adults with mild intellectual disability tend to report relatively high rates of psychological and emotional difficulties (Emerson, 2011; Ferrari, 2009; Hassiotis et al., 2008; Maughan, Collishaw and Pickles, 1999). Third, people with mild intellectual disabilities are at significantly greater risk than their peers of being exposed to common 'social determinants' of poorer mental health including childhood poverty, violence, unemployment and other forms of social exclusion (Emerson, 2007, 2012a, online early; Emerson and Jahoda, 2013; Emerson et al., 2005; Hughes et al., 2012; Jones et al., 2012).

Challenging behaviours (such as aggression, destruction and self-injury) are shown by 10–15% of people with intellectual disabilities, with age-specific prevalence peaking between the ages of 20 and 49 (Cooper et al., 2009a, 2009b; Emerson and Einfeld, 2011; Emerson et al., 2001; Holden and Gitlesen, 2006; Lowe et al., 2007; Oliver and Richards, 2010).

Dementia

The prevalence of dementia is higher amongst older adults with intellectual disabilities compared with the general population (22% vs 6% aged 65+), and is associated with a range of potentially challenging behaviours and health problems (Cooper, 1997b, 1997c; Glover et al., 2012a; Kannabiran and Deb, 2010). People with Down's syndrome are at particularly high risk of developing dementia, with the age of onset being 30–40 years younger than that for the general population (Coppus et al., 2006; Holland et al., 1998; Kannabiran and Deb, 2010).

Epilepsy

The prevalence rate of epilepsy amongst people with intellectual disabilities has been reported as at least 20 times higher than for the general population, with seizures commonly being multiple and resistant to drug treatment (Amiet et al., 2008; Arshad et al., 2011; Beange et al., 1995; Branford, Bhaumik and Duncan, 1998; Cardoza and Kerr, 2010; Glover et al., 2012a; Matthews et al., 2008; Oeseburg et al., 2011; Straetmans et al., 2007). Uncontrolled epilepsy can have serious negative consequences for both quality of life and mortality (Kerr and Bowley, 2001a, 2001b). A recent review of English-language published research found evidence of the misdiagnosis of epilepsy in people with intellectual disabilities, including both false positives and false negatives that may result in inappropriate treatment (Chapman et al., 2010). Anti-epilepsy medication is associated with a number of problems (Boyle et al., 2010), that may be greater for people with intellectual disabilities (Sipes et al., 2011).

Sleep disorders

A recent systematic review estimated prevalence rates of sleep problems in adults with intellectual disabilities ranging from 9% to 34%, with an estimated prevalence of 9% being reported for significant sleep problems (van de Wouw, Evenhuis and Echteld, 2012).

Sensory functions and pain

Sensory impairments

People with intellectual disabilities are significantly more likely to have a visual and/or hearing impairment than their non-disabled peers (Beange et al., 1995; Carvill, 2001; Das et al., 2010; Emerson and Robertson, 2011; Nielsen, Skov and Jensen, 2007a, 2007b; Oeseburg et al., 2011; van Splunder et al., 2004, 2006; Welinder and Baggesen, 2012; Woodhouse, 2010). People with Down's syndrome are at particularly high risk of developing vision and hearing loss (Beange et al., 1995; Carvill, 2001; Radhakrishnan, 2010). Carers of people with intellectual disabilities may fail to identify sensory impairments (Evenhuis, 2001; Kerr et al., 2003; Warburg, 2001).

Pain

There is an increased risk of acute and chronic pain amongst people with intellectual disabilities as a result of high rates of co-occurring health conditions and physical impairments (Oberlander et al., 2012; Symons, Shinde and Gilles, 2008). In one recent study, 67% of people with intellectual disabilities who were asked about their health reported pain, and 18% said they did not tell people when they were in pain (Turk et al., 2012). Higher rates of the experience of pain have been reported in studies of children with developmental disabilities (Breau et al., 2003; Stallard et al., 2001). When experiencing pain, children with developmental disabilities show poorer communication, daily living, social and motor skills (Breau, Camfield, McGrath and Finley, 2007). Carers may have difficulty in recognising expressions of need, or the experience of pain, particularly if the person concerned does not communicate verbally (Kerr et al., 2003; McGuire, Daly and Smyth, 2010; Purcell, Morris and McConkey, 1999).

Voice and speech functions

Communication disorders are extremely common amongst people with intellectual disabilities (McQueen et al., 1987; Pinborough-Zimmerman et al., 2007), especially more severe intellectual disability (Belva et al., 2012). Nearly 50% of children with speech and language problems are children with intellectual disability (Pinborough-Zimmerman et al., 2007). The high rates of communication disorders amongst people with intellectual disabilities have led to an extensive research programme on developing interventions to increase communication capacity (Fossett and Mirenda, 2007; Kaiser and Trent, 2007; Snell et al., 2010; Wilkinson and Hennig, 2007).

Functions of the cardiovascular, haematological, immunological and respiratory systems

Cardiovascular

Coronary heart defects and disease are a leading cause of death amongst people with intellectual disabilities (14–20%) (Hollins et al., 1998), with rates expected to rise due to increased longevity (Wells et al., 1995). Almost half of all people with Down's syndrome are affected by congenital heart defects (Brookes and Alberman, 1996; Hermon et al., 2001). It is unclear whether the overall prevalence of cardiovascular disease, including myocardial infarction and cerebrovascular accidents, amongst people with intellectual disabilities and risk factors for cardiovascular disease, differs from that seen in the general population (de Winter et al., 2012a; Department of Health, 2011; Hsu et al., 2012c; Jansen et al., 2013; Merrick and Morad, 2010; Morin et al., 2012; Oeseburg et al., 2011; Wee et al., in press).

Respiratory disease

Respiratory disease is the leading cause of death for people with intellectual disabilities (46–52%), with rates much higher than for the general population (15–17%) (Douglas, 2010; Hollins et al., 1998; Puri et al., 1995; Thillai, 2010). Higher rates of asthma, chronic obstructive pulmonary disease and upper respiratory tract infections have been reported for people with intellectual disabilities (Emerson et al., 2011a; Glover et al., 2012a; Oeseburg et al., 2011; Samele et al., 2006; Straetmans et al., 2007).

Haematological

Recent research has suggested that asymptomatic inflammation in the bloodstream of older adults with intellectual disability might contribute to their 'premature aging' (Carmeli et al., 2012).

Functions of the digestive, metabolic and endocrine Systems

Oral Health

Approximately one in three adults with intellectual disabilities have unhealthy teeth and gums (Barr et al., 1999; Fedele and Scully, 2010; Fernandez et al., 2012;

Tiller, Wilson and Gallagher, 2001). A recent UK survey involving 387 adults with intellectual disabilities reported that participants with intellectual disabilities had higher rates of untreated decay, a greater number of extractions and were less likely to have posterior functional contacts than adults in the general population (Davies, 2012). A large-scale US study based on the electronic dental records of 4732 adults with intellectual and developmental disabilities reported a prevalence of untreated caries of 32%, periodontitis of 80% and edentulism of 11% (Morgan et al., 2012).

Dysphagia
Difficulties with eating, drinking and swallowing have implications for health, safety and well-being including recurrent respiratory tract infections, asphyxia, dehydration and poor nutritional status (Chadwick and Jolliffe, 2009; Harding and Wright, 2010). Dysphagia may affect 8% of adults known to intellectual disability services (Chadwick and Jolliffe, 2009). More recent research has estimated that 15% of adults known to specialist intellectual disability services require mealtime support (Ball et al., 2012).

Gastro-oesophageal reflux disease
Gastro-oesophageal reflux disease (GORD) causes pain and may contribute to sleep disturbance, problem behaviour, anaemia and risk of oesophageal cancer (NHS Health Scotland, 2004). High rates of GORD (approximately 50%) have been reported for people with intellectual disabilities (Böhmer et al., 1999; Davis, 2010).

Constipation
Constipation has been reported amongst two-thirds of a sample of institutionalised people with moderate and severe intellectual disabilities (Böhmer et al., 2001; Davis, 2010). Although people with intellectual disabilities may be more likely to be taking drugs associated with side effects that include constipation, diagnosis of constipation is often missed due to communication problems (Coleman and Spurling, 2010).

Endocrine
Hypothyroidism is relatively common amongst people with Down's syndrome, with prevalence increasing with age. Reported prevalence rates in children with Down's syndrome range from 10 to 20% (Gibson et al., 2005; Mani, 1988; Noble et al., 2000; Pueschel, Jackson and Giesswein, 1991). A recent study has reported gradual improvements in thyroid hormone levels over a 15-year follow-up period and suggests that the incidence of hypothyroidism in people with Down's syndrome may be somewhat lower than would have been expected based on earlier prevalence studies (Prasher, Ninan and Haque, 2011). Children with profound intellectual disabilities may be at greater risk of experiencing short stature due to untreated growth hormone deficiency (Abdullah et al., 2009).

Increased rates of diabetes amongst adults with intellectual disabilities have been reported in population-based studies (Glover et al., 2012a; Reichard and Stolzle, 2011; Straetmans et al., 2007).

Genitourinary and reproductive functions

Women with intellectual disabilities experience problems with menstruation such as heavy periods, premenstrual syndrome and painful periods as often as other women. However, these problems may not be appropriately recognised by carers and may be experienced differently or more negatively (Rodgers, Lipscombe and Santer, 2006). Women with intellectual disabilities – and in particular women with Down's syndrome – tend to have earlier menopause than other women; early menopause has also been found to be associated with dementia (Coppus et al., 2010; Schupf et al., 1997). Women with intellectual disabilities may be at greater risk of adverse pregnancy and birth outcomes including greater rates of pre-eclampsia and low birth weight (McConnell, Mayes and Llewellyn, 2008).

Neuromusculoskeletal and movement-related functions

Physical impairments
Amongst adults with intellectual disabilities, mobility restrictions have been identified as significant risk factors for mortality (Tyrer and McGrother, 2009). A population-based study in the Netherlands reported that people with intellectual disabilities are 14 times more likely to have musculoskeletal impairments (van Schrojenstein Lantman De Valk et al., 2000). The prevalence of cerebral palsy amongst children with intellectual disability ranges from 8 to 34% (Oeseburg et al., 2011). The prevalence of arthritis appears to be marginally lower amongst adults with intellectual disability (Department of Health, 2011). Higher rates of sarcopenia, a syndrome characterised by progressive and generalised loss of skeletal muscle mass and strength, has been reported amongst older adults with intellectual disability (Bastiaanse et al., 2012).

Osteoporosis
People with intellectual disabilities have increased prevalence of osteoporosis and lower bone density than the general population (Center, Beange and McElduff, 1998; Department of Health, 2011; Jaffe, Timell and Gulanski, 2001; Jaffe et al., 2005; Mergler et al., 2009; Petrone, 2012; Tyler, Snyder and Zyzanski, 2000). Contributory factors include lack of weight-bearing exercise, delayed puberty, earlier-than-average age at menopause for women, poor nutrition, being underweight and use of anti-epilepsy medication. Fractures can occur with only minor injury and may be multiple (NHS Health Scotland, 2004; Petrone, 2012). Frailty amongst people with intellectual disability at age 50 to 64 is as high as in the general population aged 65 and older (Evenhuis et al., 2012).

Injuries, accidents and falls

Adults with intellectual disabilities experience higher rates of injuries and falls than their non-disabled peers (Finlayson et al., 2010; Grant, Pickett et al., 2001; Hsieh, Heller and Miller, 2001; Hsieh, Rimmer and Heller, 2012; Janicki et al., 2002; Sherrard, Tonge and Ozanne-Smith, 2002; Smulders et al., in press; Wagemans and Cluitmans, 2006).

Functions of the skin and related structures

Acne, eczema and other skin problems have been reported at higher rates amongst adults with intellectual disability (Beange et al., 1995; Schieve et al., 2012; Straetmans et al., 2007).

Cancer

The proportion of people with intellectual disabilities who die from cancer and the prevalence of cancer are lower amongst adults with intellectual disability than in the general population, although people with intellectual disabilities have proportionally higher rates of gastrointestinal cancer (Cooke, 1997; Department of Health, 2011; Duff et al., 2001; Jancar, 1990). However, the incidence and pattern of cancer amongst people with intellectual disabilities is rapidly changing due, in part, to increased longevity (Bonell, 2010; Cooke, 1997; Duff et al., 2001; Jancar, 1990). Children with Down's syndrome are at higher risk of leukaemia than other children (Hasle, Clemmensen and Mikkelsen, 2000; Hermon et al., 2001). There is a high prevalence of *Helicobacter pylori*, a class-1 carcinogen linked to stomach cancer, gastric ulcer and lymphoma amongst people with intellectual disabilities (Clarke et al., 2008; Douglas, 2010; Hogg and Tuffrey-Wijne, 2009).

Summary and conclusions

In the preceding sections we have provided a brief overview of what is known about the health of people with intellectual disabilities, with a particular focus on the differences in health status between people with and without intellectual disabilities. In many, but not all, aspects of health people with intellectual disabilities are disadvantaged when compared with their peers. In some areas (e.g. mortality, mental health, speech and communication disorders) these differences are stark. We need to keep in mind, however, that this body of evidence primarily relates to the 'visible minority' of people with more severe intellectual disabilities, who are known to specialised intellectual disability services.

We know much less about the health of the 'hidden majority' of people with mild intellectual disabilities, most of whom (as adults) are not known to specialised intellectual disability services. However, the little evidence that is available suggests that, when compared with their non-disabled peers, people with mild intellectual disabilities are more likely to: have poorer health; be exposed to social conditions detrimental to positive health; and engage in riskier health behaviours (Campbell and Fedeyko, 2001; Emerson, 2011; Snell and Luckasson, 2009; Tymchuk et al., 2001).

4

Applying a health inequalities perspective

In this chapter we will apply a broad public health perspective to understanding the health inequalities faced by people with intellectual disabilities.

Health inequalities

In Chapter 2 we provided an overview of health and some of the social determinants of health. Clearly, the influences on (or determinants of) health are complex, ranging from the influence of our genetic inheritance through the way we live (e.g. whether we smoke, drink too much, exercise too little) to the broader social and environmental conditions into which we are born, grow up and live out our lives. So too are the influences on and determinants of inequalities in health (Kreiger, 2011; Marmot and Wilkinson, 2006; Wilkinson and Pickett, 2009; World Health Organization, 2008; World Health Organization Regional Office for Europe, 2011, 2012). There are many ways of conceptualising and categorising these influences. One of the iconic frameworks is the 'rainbow model' developed by Göran Dahlgren and Margaret Whitehead in 1991 (see Figure 4.1, modified from Dahlgren and Whitehead, 1991/2007).

The model draws attention to the range of factors that shape our health, and also the interconnectedness between different 'layers' of the rainbow. So, for example, the general socio-economic, cultural and environmental conditions of any given society will have a profound impact on the living and working conditions experienced by particular groups of people in that society. Similarly, these broader 'social determinants' of health along with constitutional factors and social and community networks will shape individual lifestyle factors that are important for health (e.g. exercise, nutrition, smoking and drug use). We will use this model in this chapter to structure our consideration of the determinants of the health of (and health inequalities experienced by) people with intellectual disabilities.

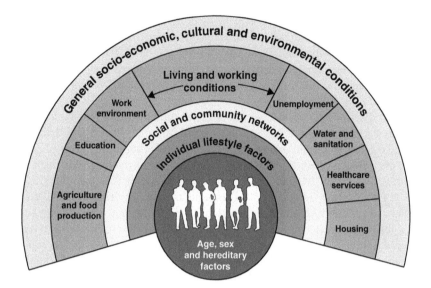

Figure 4.1 The Dahlgren and Whitehead 'rainbow model' of health determinants

Determinants of the health inequalities experienced by people with intellectual disabilities

General socio-economic, cultural and environmental conditions

Prevailing socio-economic, cultural and environmental conditions have a profound impact on shaping the material and psychosocial characteristics of our living conditions. They influence the types and quantity of food we can access, our risk of exposure to infectious diseases, the education we receive, the type and quality of housing we can afford, the types of employment that may be available to us, our opportunities for leisure activities, our security and safety, our feelings of connectedness to others and to the community in which we live, our access to social networks, and our access to timely and effective healthcare. There are, however, inequalities within all countries with regard to the ability of different groups in society (e.g. people living in poverty, people from some minority ethnic communities, people with disabilities) to access the types of living conditions that promote positive health (Australian Institute of Health and Welfare, 2012; Centers for Disease Control and Prevention (CDC), 2011; Department for Work and Pensions, 2013; Kreiger, 2011; National Equality Panel, 2010; The Marmot Review, 2010; Townsend and Davidson, 1982; World Health Organization, 2008; World Health Organization Regional Office for Europe, 2011, 2012).

Of particular relevance to understanding the health inequalities experienced by people with intellectual disabilities is the extent and pervasiveness of pejorative and discriminatory cultural attitudes about people with intellectual disability.

Such attitudes are likely to have shaped the design and operation of mainstream social institutions (e.g. education) as well as the nature of services and supports available to people with intellectual disabilities (Trent, 1994; Wolfensberger, 1975). Through their reflection in popular media, films and novels they may shape the attitudes, beliefs and actions of others (Carter, Parmenter and Watters, 2006; Chen et al., 2012; Iyer, 2007).

Whilst discriminatory attitudes about intellectual disability may be less common than a century ago, it is clear that a significant minority of people in high-income countries do hold markedly negative attitudes about the rights of people with intellectual disabilities and show unwillingness to interact with them. For example, in a recent telephone survey of 1605 randomly selected adults in the province of Québec, Canada, 40% of respondents did not think that adults with intellectual disability should have the right to drink alcohol, 30% did not think that adults with intellectual disability should have the right to have children and 25% did not think that adults with intellectual disability should have the right to walk about town unaccompanied (Morin et al., 2013). Similarly, 10% of UK adults report that they would not be comfortable interacting with a neighbour with intellectual disability (compared with 20% who reported that they *would* feel comfortable with others saying negative things about people with intellectual disabilities) (Stainland, 2011). One in three of adults in Hong Kong reported that people with intellectual disabilities should stay within their supported accommodation services, and one in six reporting that these services should be built 'far away' from residential centres (Lau and Cheung, 1999).

The importance of such beliefs is twofold. First, to the extent that they are embedded in our social institutions they restrict the access of disabled people to living conditions that are associated with better health (e.g. better education; wealth; autonomy and power; better quality housing; secure and rewarding employment; access to timely and effective healthcare) (Department for Work and Pensions, 2013; Emerson et al., 2012c, in press; House of Lords and House of Commons Joint Committee on Human Rights, 2008; World Health Organization and the World Bank, 2011). Second, members of the public that hold strong negative beliefs may be more likely to harass, abuse, bully or, in extreme cases, perpetrate violent crimes against people with intellectual disabilities (Roulstone and Mason-Bish, 2012; Sherry, 2010). Over the past twelve months 11% of UK adults with intellectual or cognitive impairments reported having been the victim of violent crime and 9% the victim of hate crime (compared with rates of 4% and 2%, respectively, amongst UK adults with no impairments) (Emerson and Roulstone, in press). As with other marginalised or 'vulnerable' groups, exposure to overt acts of disablism and violence is likely to be damaging to a person's health (Hughes et al., 2012; Krieger, 1999).

It is as a result of the growing awareness of the impact of discriminatory socio-cultural practices on constraining the life experiences of people with disabilities that disability itself is being increasingly seen as a human rights issue (Hauland and Allen, 2009; House of Lords and House of Commons Joint Committee on

Human Rights, 2008; Megret, 2008; United Nations, 2003, 2006; World Health Organization and the World Bank, 2011). As recently argued by the World Health Organization and World Bank,

> disability is a human rights issue because:
> - People with disabilities experience inequalities – for example, when they are denied equal access to healthcare, employment, education, or political participation because of their disability.
> - People with disabilities are subject to violations of dignity – for example, when they are subjected to violence, abuse, prejudice, or disrespect because of their disability.
> - Some people with disability are denied autonomy – for example, when they are subjected to involuntary sterilization, or when they are confined in institutions against their will, or when they are regarded as legally incompetent because of their disability. (World Health Organization and the World Bank, 2011)

The need to address the discrimination faced by people with disabilities (and the pervasive disablism that gives rise to such discrimination) has been highlighted in numerous reports, national legislation and the development (and ratification by the majority of the world's countries, including the UK)[1] of the UN Convention on the Rights of Persons with Disabilities (UNCRPD) (United Nations, 2006).

Article 2 of the UNCRPD defines discrimination on the basis of disability as '... any distinction, exclusion or restriction on the basis of disability which has the purpose or effect of impairing or nullifying the recognition, enjoyment or exercise, on an equal basis with others, of all human rights and fundamental freedoms in the political, economic, social, cultural, civil or any other field. It includes all forms of discrimination, including denial of reasonable accommodation'. The term disablism refers to 'the social beliefs and actions that oppress/exclude/disadvantage people with impairments' and includes consideration of both the overt and systemic (or institutional) discrimination faced by people with certain health conditions or impairments (Thomas, 2007).

In the landmark report *Death by Indifference*, Mencap defined institutional discrimination in the following terms:

> ... institutional discrimination results when organisations fail to make changes in the way they deliver their services to take into account people's differing needs. Nor does the organisation deal with ignorance and prejudice within the workforce and culture of the organisation. We believe that there is a fundamental lack of understanding and respect towards people with an intellectual disability and their families and carers. This lack of understanding

---

[1] 124 as of 21 March 2013; www.un.org/disabilities/countries.asp?id=166.

and respect leads to – and is demonstrated by – the poor design of systems, policies and procedures to meet the particular and differing needs of patients with an [intellectual] disability. (Mencap, 2007)

Living and working conditions

In the sections below, we will summarise existing evidence on the extent to which people with intellectual disabilities have access to the 'living and working conditions' that promote better health.

Exposure to social and environmental adversities

People with intellectual disabilities are more likely than their non-disabled peers to be exposed to a range of 'social determinants' of poorer health. These include poverty, poor housing conditions, unemployment, social exclusion, violence and exposure to overt acts of abuse, victimisation and discrimination (Durkin, 2002; Emerson, 2011, 2012a, online early; Emerson, Graham and Hatton, 2006a; Emerson and Hatton, 2010; Emerson and Roulstone, in press; Emerson et al., 2005, 2009, 2012c, in press; Fujiura, 1998; Harrell, 2011, 2012; Heber, 1970; Hughes et al., 2012; Jones et al., 2012; Leonard et al., 2005; Maulik et al., 2011; World Health Organization and the World Bank, 2011). To give some relatively contemporary examples:

- In 2010 English children with intellectual disabilities were twice as likely as their peers to live in poor households (Emerson, 2012a);
- Between 2001 and 2005, families with a child with intellectual disabilities in the UK were more likely to become poor and were less likely to escape from being poor than other families (Emerson et al., 2010);
- In 2003/4, 27% of 13–14-year-old English adolescents with mild to moderate intellectual disabilities who were attending mainstream school reported being bullied at least weekly (compared with 13% of children without intellectual disabilities) (Emerson et al., 2011a).
- Local authority returns for 2010/11 indicated that 7% of working-age adults with intellectual disabilities were in any form of paid employment, with just 2% of men and less than 1% of women working for 30 or more hours per week (Emerson et al., 2012b). In Victoria, Australia, 14% of adults with intellectual disability were in some form of employment compared with 61% of non-disabled adults.
- In 2009/11, UK adults with self-reported impairments of intellectual ability or understanding were nearly three times more likely than their non-disabled peers to have been a victim of violent crime over the previous year and nearly seven times more likely to have been a victim of hate crime (Emerson and Roulstone, in press).
- Over the same period, whilst rates of violent crime victimisation were marginally declining in the USA (from 2.3% to 2.0% per year), violent crime victimisation of adults with cognitive impairments rose from 4.6% to 5.1% (Harrell, 2012).

Given the association between minority ethnic status and poverty, and the exposure of people with intellectual disabilities from minority ethnic communities to overt racism (Azmi et al., 1997; Mir et al., 2004), it is likely that people with intellectual disabilities from minority ethnic communities will face greater health inequalities than people with intellectual disabilities from majority ethnic communities.

This increased risk of exposure to environmental adversities amongst people with intellectual disabilities is the result of a number of different factors that vary in their importance across the life course (Emerson et al., 2012c, in press). These include the following.

- Exposure to some adversities (e.g. child poverty) is known to impair cognitive development and will consequently increase the risk of the development of (especially mild) intellectual disabilities (Duncan and Brooks-Gunn, 2000; Duncan, Brooks-Gunn and Klebanov, 1994; Shonkoff, 2010; Shonkoff, Boyce and McEwen, 2009).
- Discrimination experienced by people with intellectual disabilities is likely to constrain their life opportunities and increase the risk of poverty and social exclusion, as well as exposure to incidents of overt discrimination and abuse (see above).
- The additional direct (e.g. costs associated with travel to appointments, additional healthcare expenditure) and indirect costs (e.g. reduced maternal employment) associated with supporting a person with intellectual disability may increase the risk of becoming poor and reduce the chances of escaping from poverty (Emerson et al., 2010; Parish and Cloud, 2006; Parish et al., 2008; Shahtahmasebi et al., 2011).
- Some parental/family factors (e.g. low parental intelligence, maternal alcohol abuse) may be associated with both increasing the risk of their children developing intellectual disabilities and of becoming poor (IASSID Special Interest Research Group on Parents and Parenting with Intellectual Disabilities, 2008).

Whatever the underlying reasons, exposure to these types of adversities is predictive of poorer well-being amongst people with intellectual disabilities, with the strength of the association appearing to be at least as strong as it is amongst the general population (Dickson, Emerson and Hatton, 2005; Emerson, 2010; Emerson and Einfeld, 2010; Emerson and Hatton, 2007a, 2007b, 2007c; Emerson et al., 2010, 2011b;). As such, we would expect that people with intellectual disabilities would have poorer health, not because of their intellectual disability per se but because they are more likely than their non-disabled peers to be exposed to a range of 'social determinants' of poorer health.

This is an issue we have been researching over the last decade. Our results suggest that increased exposure to low socio-economic position/poverty may account for:

- 20–50% of the increased risk for poorer physical and mental health amongst UK children and adolescents with intellectual disabilities (Emerson and Hatton, 2007a, 2007b, 2007c);

- 29–43% of the increased risk for conduct difficulties and 36–43% of the increased risk for peer problems amongst Australian children with intellectual disabilities or borderline intellectual functioning (Emerson et al., 2010);
- a significant proportion of increased rates of self-reported antisocial behaviour amongst adolescents with intellectual disabilities (Dickson et al., 2005; Emerson and Halpin, 2013);
- 32% of the increased risk for conduct difficulties and 27% of the increased risk for peer problems amongst a nationally representative sample of 3-year-old UK children with developmental delay (Emerson and Einfeld, 2010);
- All of the increased self-reported risk of fighting/public disturbance, shoplifting and graffiti writing amongst adolescents with intellectual disability (Emerson and Halpin, 2013).

It is important to note that *all* of the research listed above has been undertaken on population-based samples of children or youth with intellectual disability, in which the vast majority of children have mild/moderate intellectual disability. Research relating to the association between exposure to low socio-economic position (and associated environmental adversities), and the well-being of adults with intellectual disability or people with severe intellectual disabilities is more limited and more complex given: (1) the difficulty of measuring socio-economic position (SEP) amongst adults with intellectual disability when attainment on most indicators of SEP (e.g. educational attainment, income, employment status) is uniformly low; and (2) the questionable validity of using locality-based measures of deprivation as a proxy for SEP for people living in supported accommodation arrangements (Emerson, Graham and Hatton, 2006b; Emerson and Hatton, 2010).

Indeed, the results of research on the association between SEP (and associated environmental adversities) and the well-being of adults with intellectual disability are rather mixed. A small number of studies focusing on adults with predominantly mild intellectual disabilities have reported significant associations between low SEP and poorer self-rated health (Emerson and Hatton, 2008c), lower self-reported well-being (Emerson and Hatton, 2008b), poorer mental health (Emerson and Brigham, unpublished) and riskier health behaviours (Emerson and Brigham, unpublished). Figure 4.2, for example, illustrates the clear dose-dependent relationship between breadth of exposure to five indicators of low SEP (major wage earner unemployed, low income, poor housing, temporary accommodation, three or more changes of address in the previous year) and Health Visitor assessments of alcohol and drug abuse, smoking and poor mental health amongst parents with intellectual disability in South West England.

Amongst adults with intellectual disabilities more generally there exists a modest, but expanding, literature on the association between exposure to potentially adverse life events and poorer mental health (Cooper et al., 2007a, 2007b; Esbensen and Benson, 2006; Hamilton, Sutherland and Iacono, 2005; Hastings et al., 2004; Hulbert-Williams and Hastings, 2008; Murphy, O'Callaghan and Clare, 2007; Owen et al., 2004; Sequeira and Hollins, 2003), including amongst people with profound intellectual disability (Cooper et al., 2007a). The importance of this literature is that risk exposure to life events is predicted by SEP and is likely to be one

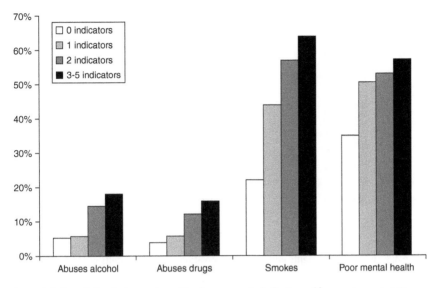

Figure 4.2 Association between breadth of exposure to indicators of low socio-economic position (SEP) and health behaviours and mental health of parents with intellectual disability

of the mediating pathways that links SEP to poorer health (Emerson and Jahoda, 2013).

However, other studies have failed to find associations between poorer mental health or challenging behaviours and indicators of low SEP (such as locality-based measures of deprivation and unemployment) or life events (Cooper et al., 2007a, 2007b, 2009a, 2009b; Gray et al., 2012; Reid, Smiley and Cooper, 2011). As mentioned above, the use of locality-based measures of neighbourhood deprivation as a proxy measure for individual- or household-level SEP can be problematic for adults with intellectual disability who are living in supported accommodation arrangements (Emerson and Hatton, 2010; Emerson et al., 2006b), although they remain valid as indicators of neighbourhood deprivation per se. Figure 4.3, for example, shows the percentage of adults with intellectual disability in England living in the two least deprived and two most deprived quintiles of neighbourhood deprivation. As can be seen, adults living in supported accommodation are less likely than those living independently or with their families to be living in more deprived areas and more likely to be living in less deprived areas.

There is a clear need for future research to investigate the significance of exposure to social determinants of health in accounting for the health inequalities faced by people with intellectual disabilities and how this may vary with such factors as age, gender, ethnicity, severity of intellectual disability and syndromes associated with intellectual disability. For example, Figure 4.4 shows the association between breadth of exposure to indicators of low SEP and associated adversities at age 9 months and 3 years, and persistence of conduct difficulties from age 3 to ages 5 and 7 amongst typically developing UK children, children with intellectual

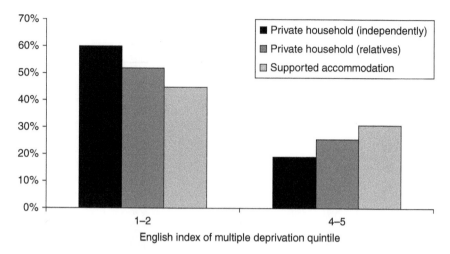

Figure 4.3 Living arrangements and locality deprivation for English adults with intellectual disability, 2003/4

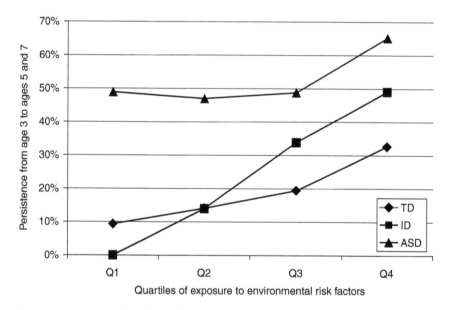

Figure 4.4 Persistence of conduct difficulties at age 5 and 7 years by child impairment and breadth of exposure to adversities at age 9 months and 3 years

disability who do not have autism spectrum disorder and children with autism spectrum disorder (Emerson et al., unpublished). As can be seen, for both typically developing children and those with intellectual disability who do not have autism spectrum disorder there is a clear association between breadth of exposure to adversity in the early years and the persistence of conduct difficulties across middle childhood. However, no such association is apparent for children with autism spectrum disorder.

Access to, and the quality of, healthcare and other services

Considerable attention has been drawn over the last decade to the importance of inequalities in relation to one key aspect of the general 'living and working conditions' experienced by people with intellectual disabilities: whether they have timely access to appropriate and effective healthcare (Disability Rights Commission, 2006; Heslop et al., 2013; House of Lords and House of Commons Joint Committee on Human Rights, 2008; Krahn and Fox, in press; Krahn et al., 2006; Mencap, 2007, 2012a; Michael, 2008; US Department of Health and Human Services, 2002a, 2002b). This is likely to be a particularly important issue for people with intellectual disabilities from indigenous or minority ethnic groups (Hatton et al., 1998, 2003; Magana et al., 2012).

A range of barriers to accessing healthcare services have been identified (Alborz, McNally and Glendinning, 2005; Alborz, McNally and Swallow, 2003; Allerton and Emerson, online early; Dinsmore, 2011; Disability Rights Commission, 2006; Giraud-Saunders, 2009; Heslop et al., 2013; Krahn and Fox, in press; Krahn et al., 2006; Kwok and Cheung, 2007; Lagu et al., 2013; McInnis, Hills and Chapman, 2011; Michael, 2008; Norwood and Slayton, 2013; O'Hara, 2010; Owens, Dyer and Mistry, 2010; Rippon, 2010; Schieve et al., 2012; Turk et al., 2010; US Department of Health and Human Services, 2002a, 2002b). These include:

- scarcity of appropriate services;
- inability to afford services;
- delays in access to care, diagnosis and treatment;
- physical and informational barriers to access;
- unhelpful, inexperienced or discriminatory healthcare staff;
- failure of healthcare providers to make 'reasonable adjustments' in light of the literacy and communication difficulties experienced by many people with intellectual disabilities;
- 'diagnostic overshadowing' (e.g. symptoms of physical ill health being mistakenly attributed to either a mental health/behavioural problem or as being inherent in the person's intellectual disabilities).

Particular concern has been expressed about the risks faced by people with intellectual disabilities (and especially those who also show 'challenging behaviour') when detained in institutional settings (Care Quality Commission, 2012; Department of Health, 2012b, 2012c; Emerson, 2012b; Glover and Olson, 2012; Mencap and Challenging Behaviour Foundation, 2012; World Health Organization Regional

Office for Europe, 2010a). These include concerns about the inappropriate medical treatment of people with intellectual disabilities with 'challenging behaviour' such as high rates of off-label prescription of anti-psychotic medication (de Kuijper et al., 2010; Department of Health, 2007; Emerson et al., 2000; Kiernan, Reeves and Alborz, 1995; Molyneux, Emerson and Caine, 1999; Robertson et al., 2000a, 2005; Royal College of Psychiatrists, British Psychological Society and Royal College of Speech and Language Therapists, 2007; Straetmans et al., 2007; Tsiouris, 2010). This is of concern as: (1) there is little evidence that anti-psychotics have any specific effect in reducing challenging behaviours; and (2) such medication has a number of well-documented serious side effects (Emerson and Einfeld, 2011; Mencap and Challenging Behaviour Foundation, 2012; Tsiouris, 2010).

In the following sections we summarise knowledge about inequalities in access to: health screening and health promotion; primary healthcare; and secondary healthcare.

Health screening and health promotion
A number of studies have reported low uptake of health promotion or screening activities amongst people with intellectual disabilities (Alborz et al., 2003, 2005; Jensen, Taylor and Davis, in press). These include:

- assessment for vision or hearing impairments (Lavis, Cullen and Roy, 1997; McGlade et al., 2010; Woodhouse, 2010; Woodhouse et al., 2012; Yeates, 1995);
- routine dental care (Barr et al., 1999; Emerson et al., 2005; Fernandez et al., 2012; Norwood and Slayton, 2013; Owens et al., 2010);
- cervical smear tests (Department of Health, 2011; Djuretic et al., 1999; Glover et al., 2012a; Morgan et al., 2012; Osborn et al., 2012; Pearson et al., 1998; Reynolds, Stanistreet and Elton, 2008);
- breast self-examinations and mammography (Davies and Duff, 2001; Department of Health, 2011; Djuretic et al., 1999; Glover et al., 2012a; Osborn et al., 2012; Piachaud and Rohde, 1998; Truesdale-Kennedy, Taggart and McIlfatrick, 2011; Willis et al., 2008);
- bowel and prostate screening (Department of Health, 2011; Osborn et al., 2012).

Access to health promotion may be significantly poorer for people with more severe intellectual disabilities (Kerr, Felce and Felce, 2005) and people with intellectual disabilities who do not use intellectual disability services (Emerson, 2011). There is some evidence that access to screening may vary by level of neighbourhood deprivation, though the direction of effects is somewhat inconsistent (Cooper et al., 2011). Staff in residential care homes may have insufficient training and skills to effectively engage people with intellectual disabilities in health-promotion activities and/or to have access to important relevant information such as a person's family history (Hanna, Taggart and Cousins, 2011).

Primary healthcare

There is conflicting evidence on whether people with intellectual disabilities make more or less use of primary healthcare services than their non-disabled peers (Kerr, Richards and Glover, 1996; Piachaud, Rohde and Pasupathy, 1998; Stein and Ball, 1999; Straetmans et al., 2007; Turk et al., 2010; Whitfield, Langan and Russell, 1996). However, given the evidence (see above) of greater health needs, it would be expected that people with intellectual disabilities should be accessing primary care services more frequently than the general population. For example, comparison of general practitioner consultation rates to those of patients with other chronic conditions suggests that primary care access rates for people with intellectual disabilities are lower than might be expected (Felce et al., 2008b). In a recent study, mean consultation rates for adults with intellectual disabilities were found to be lower than for the general population; increased age, female gender and having a paid carer were associated with greater use of GP services (Turk et al., 2010).

Collaboration between GPs, primary healthcare teams and specialist services for people with intellectual disabilities is generally regarded as poor (Thornton, 1999). Adults aged over 60 with intellectual disabilities are less likely to receive a range of health services compared with younger adults with intellectual disabilities (Cooper, 1997a).

A number of papers draw attention to the benefits of health screening to help identify unmet health needs (Jones et al., 2010; Lennox et al., 2007, 2010, 2011; McGlade et al., 2010; Robertson, Roberts and Emerson, 2010). The introduction of special health checks for people with intellectual disabilities has been shown to be effective in identifying unmet health needs, suggesting that health checks represent a 'reasonable adjustment' to the difficulties in identifying and/or communicating health need experienced by people with intellectual disabilities (Robertson et al., 2010). This has led to the introduction in England and Wales of schemes to provide financial incentives to primary care physicians to provide annual health checks for adults with intellectual disabilities (Glover, Emerson and Evison, 2012b).

Evidence of the failure of primary care services to appropriately support people with intellectual disabilities can be inferred from evidence that people with intellectual disabilities are significantly more likely to be admitted into hospital for the treatment of ambulatory care-sensitive conditions (Balogh et al., 2010, 2013; Glover and Evison, 2013). Ambulatory care-sensitive conditions are health conditions (such as constipation) that under ordinary circumstances should be managed in primary care or outpatient visits. There is evidence that people with intellectual disabilities living in more disadvantaged communities are more likely to be admitted for ambulatory care-sensitive conditions (Balogh et al., 2013).

Secondary healthcare

People with intellectual disabilities have made increased use of secondary healthcare services (Hsu et al., 2012a; Morgan, Ahmed and Kerr, 2000), including ambulatory care (Hsu et al., 2012a) and emergency department visits (Lunsky et al., 2012). A recent study has reported that people with intellectual disabilities living in areas with higher levels of deprivation made less use of secondary outpatient care but more use of accident and emergency care than those living in less deprived areas (Cooper et al., 2011).

People with intellectual disabilities and cancer are less likely to be informed of their diagnosis and prognosis, be given pain relief, be involved in decisions about their care and receive palliative care (Bernal, 2008; Tuffrey-Wijne et al., 2010; Tuffrey-Wijne, Hogg and Curfs, 2007). Concern has been expressed with regard to the availability of and access to mental health services by people with intellectual disabilities (Beecham et al., 2002; Hassiotis, Barron and O'Hara, 2000; Roy, Martin and Wells, 1997).

Social and community networks

There is extensive evidence to suggest that people who have more extensive and closer social networks and people who report feeling connected to their local community tend to have better health (Almedom, 2005; House, Landis and Umberson, 1988; Kawachi and Berkman, 2000; Murayama, Fujiwara and Kawachi, 2012; Seeman, 1996; Stansfeld, 2006; Uchino, 2006; Uchino, Cacioppo and Kiecolt-Glaser, 1996). Similar associations have been reported for people with intellectual disabilities, particularly in relation to the extent of contact with friends with intellectual disabilities (Emerson and Hatton, 2008b, 2008c; Emerson and McVilly, 2004; Emerson et al., 2005; Robertson et al., 2001; Shattuck et al., 2011). It is of concern, therefore, that people with intellectual disabilities often have highly restricted social networks (Bigby, 2008; Department of Health, 2011; Emerson and McVilly, 2004; Emerson et al., 2005; Forrester-Jones et al., 2006; Margalit, 2004; Robertson et al., 2001; Rosen and Burchard, 1990; Shephard-Jones, Prout and Kleinert, 2005; Stancliffe, 2007), in part due to being placed in educational and residential services geographically distant from their home communities (Audit Commission, 2007; Emerson and Robertson, 2008; Mencap, 2012b).

For example, results from the 2003/4 national survey of the life experiences of adults with intellectual disabilities in England indicated that (Emerson et al., 2005):

- 58% of adults with intellectual disabilities had infrequent contact with their families (compared with just 9% of adults without intellectual disabilities);
- 31% of adults with intellectual disabilities had no contact with friends (compared with just 3% of adults without intellectual disabilities);
- The most commonly reported barriers to having more social contact were:
  - living too far away or problems with travelling (44%);
  - not enough time (21%);
  - lack of money (13%);
  - not always enough support (11%);

- cannot get out or too ill (4%);
- afraid of going out (4%).

Individual lifestyle factors

Diet

Less than 10% of adults with intellectual disabilities in supported accommodation in England eat a balanced diet, with an insufficient intake of fruit and vegetables (Robertson et al., 2000b). Carers generally have poor knowledge about public-health recommendations on dietary intake (Melville et al., 2009). A large-scale population survey in Victoria, Australia, reported that: (1) 48% of adults with an intellectual disability met the recommended minimum daily intake levels for fruit, a similar percentage to adults in the general Victorian population (48%); (2) 11% of adults with an intellectual disability met the recommended minimum daily intake for vegetables, again a similar percentage to the general Victorian population (8%); and (3) 45% of adults with an intellectual disability were reported to drink water usually when thirsty, lower than the general Victorian population (73%) (Department of Health, 2011).

Exercise

Over 80% of adults with intellectual disabilities engage in levels of physical activity below the minimum recommended level, a much lower level than the general population (53–64%) (Bartlo and Klein, 2011; Department of Health, 2011; Emerson, 2005a; Messent, Cooke and Long, 1998; Robertson et al., 2000b; Wee et al., in press). People with more severe intellectual disabilities and those living in more restrictive environments are at increased risk of inactivity (Robertson et al., 2000b). In a recent study about carer intentions, only 56% of care staff planned to encourage physical activity in those they supported (Martin et al., 2011).

Obesity and underweight

People with intellectual disabilities are much more likely to be either underweight or obese than the general population (Bell and Bhate, 1992; Bhaumik et al., 2008; Choi et al., 2012; de Winter et al., 2012b; Department of Health, 2011; Dias et al., in press; Emerson, 2005a, 2009; Glover et al., 2012a; Melville et al., 2007, 2008; Messent et al., 1998; Robertson et al., 2000b; Slevin et al., in press). Globally, particularly high rates of obesity amongst people with intellectual disabilities have been reported in North America (Lloyd, Temple and Foley, 2012; Temple, Foley and Lloyd, in press). Women, people with Down's syndrome, people of higher ability, people living in less restrictive environments and women living in more deprived areas are at increased risk of obesity (Bhaumik et al., 2008; Emerson, 2005a; Melville et al., 2007, 2008; Prasher, 1995; Robertson et al., 2000b; Stancliffe et al., 2012).

Substance use

There is relatively little reliable information on the rates of substance abuse amongst people with intellectual disabilities, especially the 'hidden majority' of people with intellectual disabilities (Chapman and Wu, 2012; McGillicuddy, 2006b). The available evidence suggests that: (1) fewer adults with intellectual disabilities who use intellectual disability services smoke tobacco or drink alcohol compared with the general population (Department of Health, 2011; Fidler, Michell and Charlton, 1992; Glover et al., 2012a; Robertson et al., 2000b); (2) rates of smoking are considerably higher amongst adolescents with mild intellectual disabilities (Emerson and Turnbull, 2005), parents with intellectual disability (Emerson and Brigham, unpublished) and amongst people with intellectual disabilities who do not use intellectual disability services (Emerson, 2011); (3) there may be higher rates of substance abuse amongst people with intellectual disabilities who are substance users (Chapman and Wu, 2012; Emerson and Brigham, unpublished); and (4) people with intellectual disabilities with identified substance misuse were most likely to misuse alcohol (Chapman and Wu, 2012; Taggart et al., 2006).

Sexual health

Little is known about inequalities in the sexual health status of people with intellectual disabilities. There is, however, evidence to suggest that they may face particular barriers in accessing sexual health services and the informal channels through which young people learn about sex and sexuality (Fraser and Sim, 2007). A population-based study in the Netherlands reported that men with intellectual disabilities were eight times more likely to have sexually transmitted diseases (van Schrojenstein Lantman De Valk et al., 2000).

Constitutional factors

People with moderate to profound intellectual disabilities are more likely than the general population to die from congenital abnormalities (Tyrer and McGrother, 2009). In addition, a number of syndromes associated with intellectual disabilities are also associated with some specific health risks (Arron et al., 2011; Batshaw, Pellegrino and Roizen, 2007; Dykens, Hodapp and Finucane, 2000; Emerson and Einfeld, 2011; Harris, 2005; Jacobson et al., 2010; McCarthy et al., 2010; Melville et al., 2005; Proto et al., 2007; Stinton, Elison and Howlin, 2010; Stinton, Tomlinson and Estes, 2012; Torr and Lee, 2010). For example:

- Congenital heart disease is more prevalent amongst people with Down's syndrome and Williams syndrome.
- Early-onset dementia and immune system disorders are more common in people with Down's syndrome (Torr and Lee, 2010).
- Hypothalamic disorders are more prevalent amongst people with Prader–Willi syndrome.
- Mental health problems and challenging behaviours are more prevalent amongst people with autism spectrum disorders, Rett syndrome, Cornelia

de Lange syndrome, Riley–Day syndrome, Fragile-X syndrome, Prader–Willi syndrome, velocardiofacial syndrome /22q11.2 deletion, Williams syndrome, Lesch–Nyhan syndrome, Cri du Chat syndrome and Smith–Magenis syndrome.

- Obesity is more prevalent amongst people with Prader–Willi syndrome, Cohen syndrome, Down's syndrome and Bardet–Biedl syndrome;
- Sleep problems are more prevalent amongst children with Williams syndrome and Down's syndrome (Annaz et al., 2011; Carter et al., 2009).

In addition, approximately 33% of adults with severe or profound intellectual disabilities and 60–65% of children have difficulties of urinary incontinence and 25% have difficulties of bowel incontinence, difficulties that without effective management are associated with additional health risks (Cooper et al., 2009b; Van Laecke, 2008).

People with intellectual disabilities may have poor bodily awareness and a minority may have depressed pain responses (Gilbert-McLeod et al., 2000; March, 1991; Symons et al., 2008). In addition, limited communication skills may reduce their capacity to convey identified health needs effectively to others (e.g. relatives, friends, paid support workers). As a result, carers (unpaid and paid) play an important role in the identification of health needs for many people with more severe intellectual disabilities. However, carers may have difficulty in recognising expressions of need, or the experience of pain, particularly if the person concerned does not communicate verbally (Kerr et al., 2003; McGuire et al., 2010; Purcell, Morris and McConkey, 1999). In a recent study, 67% of people with intellectual disabilities who were asked about their health reported pain, and 18% said they did not tell people when they were in pain (Turk et al., 2012).

With regard to health literacy, whilst people with less severe intellectual disabilities may have an understanding of such issues as what it means to be healthy, have a healthy diet, the dangers of substance misuse and the benefits of exercise, they may lack knowledge in specific areas (including of healthcare) and face a range of barriers to engaging in more healthy lifestyles (Caton et al., 2012; Hawkins and Look, 2006; Jobling and Cuskelly, 2006; Parish et al., 2012; Rodgers, 1998). Care workers may feel that they do not have the knowledge, skills and training required to recognise emerging health problems or the resources to effectively promote health literacy (Hanna et al., 2011; Willis, Wishart and Muir, 2010). Information and support such as that related to breast cancer and mammography may not meet the needs of some people with intellectual disabilities (Truesdale-Kennedy et al., 2011).

Conclusions

People with intellectual disabilities are disadvantaged at every layer of Dahlgren and Whitehead's 'rainbow model' of the determinants of health (and health inequalities). In Gloria Krahn's terms, they are subject to a cascade of disparities (Krahn and Fox, in press; Krahn et al., 2006). Given the multiple and overlapping disadvantages faced by people with intellectual disabilities, it is no surprise that they experience poorer health than their non-disabled peers. This evidence also suggests that ameliorating the health inequalities faced by people with intellectual disabilities will require action at different levels of the determinants of the health 'rainbow', an issue to which we will turn in the next chapter.

5

Addressing the health inequalities faced by people with intellectual disabilities

As the previous chapters have demonstrated, people with intellectual disabilities face extensive and pervasive inequalities in health, across the life course and across a wide range of health conditions. It is also clear that much of this pervasive disadvantage in terms of health can be accounted for by the same types of social and economic determinants that apply to the rest of the population. This chapter applies a public health perspective to consider the range of strategies potentially available to address the health inequalities experienced by people with intellectual disabilities. We then review existing evidence concerning the effectiveness of health improvement strategies designed to improve the health of people with intellectual disabilities through this public health lens.

Public health perspectives on improving health and reducing health inequalities

The evidence we have reviewed so far has pointed strongly to the importance of factors far beyond specialist or generic health services when considering determinants of the health of people with intellectual disabilities. A similarly broad perspective is needed when considering how the health of people with intellectual disabilities may be improved and how the health inequalities experienced by people with intellectual disabilities can be reduced or eliminated – in other words, a public health perspective. Although the discipline and practice of public health resists easy definition, one typical definition 'the fulfillment of society's interest in assuring the conditions in which people can be healthy' (IoM, 1988) emphasises the breadth of scope of public health activity.

Disability and public health communities have until recently taken relatively little interest in each other. Historically, disability activists have been wary of aspects of public health activity such as the emphasis placed on prevention strategies, which some disability activists have interpreted as aimed at the long-term eradication of disabled people. For the purposes of this chapter, we will not be describing 'primary prevention' strategies aimed at reducing the incidence of intellectual disabilities (Emerson et al., 2011d), as we are focusing on strategies to improve the health of people with intellectual disabilities. Instead we will be focusing on 'secondary prevention' strategies designed to stop the development of health problems amongst people with intellectual disabilities, and 'tertiary' prevention strategies designed to effectively treat and/or manage already existing health problems amongst people with intellectual disabilities (Emerson et al., 2011d). However, the boundaries between these categorisations of prevention strategies are fuzzy at best. In this book so far we have contended that the nature of intellectual disability itself is socially situated, and we have provided evidence that the health of people with intellectual disabilities is subject to a broad range of socio-economic determinants. It is therefore possible that public health strategies aimed at improving the socio-economic environments within which people with intellectual disabilities live could have the dual effect of improving the health of people with intellectual disabilities, and over time reducing the number of people meeting a classification of intellectual disability.

Recently, there has been an increasing willingness of disability communities to recognise the potential contribution of public health to identifying, understanding and addressing the health inequalities experienced by disabled people, and an increasing recognition by some in the public health community that disability may be relevant to fully understanding and improving population health (Drum, Krahn and Bersani, 2009; Krahn and Campbell, 2011; Scheepers et al., 2005).

Numerous frameworks and taxonomies to organise our understanding of the range and diversity of public health activities have been developed. A recent framework, useful for understanding the range of ways in which public health may have an impact on population health, the health impact pyramid (Frieden, 2010), is presented in Figure 5.1. As Frieden explains in regard to the health impact pyramid:

> Efforts to address socio-economic determinants are at the base, followed by public health interventions that change the context for health (e.g. clean water, safe roads), protective interventions with long-term benefits (e.g. immunisations), direct clinical care, and, at the top, counselling and education. In general, public action and interventions represented by the base of the pyramid require less individual effort and have the greatest population impact … Interventions at the top tiers are designed to help individuals rather than entire populations … however, even the best programs at the pyramid's higher levels achieve limited public health impact, largely because of their dependence on long-term individual behavior change.

Whilst the correspondences are not exact, the top of the health impact pyramid is broadly consistent with actions to address the innermost rings of Dahlgren and Whitehead's rainbow model of health (age, sex and hereditary factors; individual lifestyle factors), and dropping down through the layers of the health impact pyramid is broadly equivalent to moving through the outermost rings of Dahlgren and

Whitehead's rainbow (social and community networks; general socio-economic, cultural and environmental conditions).

This health impact pyramid has a number of advantages when considering efforts to improve the health of people with intellectual disabilities. First, it explicitly takes a perspective on health improvement that separates health impact from health services, emphasising the range of actions available to address the social determinants of health that have such an impact on the health of people with intellectual disabilities. For example, recent substantial improvements from 1990 to 2007 in child mortality, maternal and child health, and health inequalities in Brazil have been achieved through a combination of healthcare reforms (to a universal, decentralised health system) allied to improvements in the education of girls, reductions in income inequalities, and improvements in water and sanitation (Barros et al., 2010).

As Frieden recognises, however, such actions can seem very remote from a 'health' agenda even though they may have significant public health impacts (e.g. action to reduce disability hate crime or reduce family poverty), and '... because these actions may address social and economic structures of society, they can be more controversial, particularly if the public does not see such interventions as falling within the government's appropriate sphere of action' (Frieden, 2010).

Second, it identifies many potentially high-impact public health approaches (particularly towards the base of the pyramid) that involve changing people's circumstances and environments in ways that improve population health but do not require the active sign-up and informed consent of individuals. Requiring informed consent or adopting complex best-interest procedures with the subgroup of people with intellectual disabilities who lack the capacity to demonstrate informed consent to health interventions may act as barriers to the implementation of health interventions that have the potential to improve the health of the entire population of people with intellectual disabilities.

Third, the separation of actions to improve population health from health services allows us to consider the potential impact of public health actions on the large proportion of adults with intellectual disabilities who are not known to specialist intellectual disability services. For illustrative purposes, we have added to Figure 5.1 a band at the bottom of the health impact pyramid, where the width of the base of the pyramid represents the population of England (approximately 51.8 million people). The darkest section on the left represents the estimated proportion of the English population who are people with intellectual disabilities known to specialist services, approximately 236,000 people or 0.5% of the population (Emerson et al., 2011e). The next section to the right adds the estimated proportion of people with intellectual disabilities not known to specialist services, another 807,000 people or 1.6% of the population (Emerson et al., 2011e). The next section adds the estimated proportion of disabled people in England minus the number of estimated people with intellectual disabilities, approximately 8.5 million people or 16.3% of the population (ODI, 2011).

We have added these figures to highlight the dilemmas involved when considering public health approaches to people with intellectual disabilities. From these figures it is easy to see why public health specialists concerned with the health of total populations forget the health needs of people with intellectual disabilities, particularly given the effective segregation of many people with intellectual disabilities within specialist services and the invisibility of intellectual disability amongst those adults with intellectual disabilities who are not known to specialist services. However, we have seen throughout this book the pervasive, extensive and preventable health inequalities experienced by people with intellectual disabilities compared with the rest of the population. In terms of improving the health of people with intellectual disabilities and reducing these health inequalities, are public health resources most effective when targeted specifically at people with intellectual disabilities (either known to specialist services or not), targeted across disability groups or designed for the general population where people with intellectual disabilities are included?

The UK is typical of many high-income countries in having disability equality legislation such as the Equality Act (Government Equalities Office, 2010), with an accompanying legal duty for all public sector services to make 'reasonable adjustments' to the manner in which they make their services available to disabled people to make them as accessible and effective as they would be for people without disabilities. Reasonable adjustments (or 'accommodations' in the language of the UN Convention on the Rights of Persons with Disabilities) include removing physical barriers to accessing health services, but importantly also include making whatever alterations are necessary to policies, procedures, staff training and service delivery to ensure that they work equally well for people with disabilities, including intellectual disabilities (Hatton, Roberts and Baines, 2011). However, reasonable adjustments are rarely routinely applied to public health approaches, and many public health actions fail to be inclusive of people with intellectual disabilities.

Finally, it is important to note that the effectiveness of public health interventions can be judged against several criteria. For example, an obvious criterion would be that the intervention improves the health of people with intellectual disabilities. However, general population interventions often preferentially benefit particular segments of the population, often the more wealthy and powerful (Lorenc et al., 2013; White, Adams and Heywood, 2009). As such they might result in smaller improvements for people with intellectual disabilities compared with other groups, resulting in worsening health inequalities. Given the health inequalities already experienced by people with intellectual disabilities, an additional criterion for public health interventions should be that they reduce the health inequalities experienced by people with intellectual disabilities compared with the rest of the population.

The rest of this chapter will examine each level of the health impact pyramid in turn, and where possible discuss evidence concerning public health interventions that are intellectual disability-specific, pan-disability- or general population-oriented, in terms of their inclusion of and impact on people with intellectual disabilities.

Level 1: counselling and education

Interventions at this level are designed to educate and/or counsel individuals to engage in more healthy behaviours. Examples of such health education and counselling interventions target behavioural change in terms of improving dietary intake, increasing physical activity, reducing alcohol intake, stopping smoking and engaging in less risky sexual behaviour (Frieden, 2010).

Diet, physical activity and weight reduction

Much of the published research concerning public health interventions specifically designed for people with intellectual disabilities has involved some variety of health promotion targeted at adults with intellectual disabilities known to specialist services. From a public health perspective this might seem somewhat paradoxical. Adults with intellectual disabilities known to specialist services are less likely to be able to provide the informed consent required for these interventions compared with people with intellectual disabilities not known to specialist services.

They are also likely to have a particular profile of health risks (see Chapters 2 and 4); although risks of obesity, low physical activity and poor diet are likely to be higher than the general population for both groups of adults with intellectual disabilities, the relatively restrictive environments of specialist services are associated with lower (although variable) rates of alcohol and substance misuse, smoking and risky sexual behaviour compared with the general population. Adults with intellectual disabilities not known to specialist services, however, are more likely to live in the disadvantaged socio-economic conditions associated with higher rates of alcohol and substance misuse, smoking and risky sexual behaviour compared with the general population. Despite the likely increased health risks of this population, they are invisible to both specialist intellectual disability services (where targeted public health interventions for people with intellectual disabilities are likely to occur) and public health interventions aimed at the general population (where these interventions often struggle to effectively reach disadvantaged populations and are not designed to be accessible to people with intellectual disabilities).

Several studies have designed and evaluated health promotion interventions designed to improve physical activity and nutrition amongst adults with intellectual disabilities known to specialist services. A scoping review (Heller et al., 2011) of 12 studies from 1986 to 2006 reported that methodological limitations in many of these studies (e.g. small sample sizes, lack of control group, lack of follow-up evaluation, multi-component programmes, lack of measurement of physical health outcomes) made it difficult to provide conclusive evidence concerning the effectiveness of these programmes in improving nutrition and physical activity. However, they did conclude that there was some promising evidence for short-term improvements in health-related attitudes and behaviours.

More recent studies have improved our understanding of the effectiveness of such health promotion programmes. For example, Wu et al. (2010) used a pre–post design to investigate the effectiveness of a physical fitness programme on weight, body mass index (BMI) and physical fitness amongst 146 institutionalised adults with intellectual disabilities over six months. This study reported improvements in weight, BMI and some measures of physical fitness over the six months, with greater effectiveness amongst more able people with intellectual disabilities than less able people with intellectual disabilities. A small (total $n = 45$) randomised controlled trial (RCT) of a 20-week exercise training intervention in adults with intellectual disabilities reported a pre–post intervention positive impact of a combined exercise training programme compared with an endurance exercise training programme and a control group on a range of indicators of physical fitness (Calders et al., 2011). A two-year follow-up evaluation of a community-based health promotion programme for 192 adults with intellectual disabilities reported reduced participation in the programme over time (often due to clashes with the routines of specialist intellectual disability services) and no overall improvement in BMI over 2 years, with around a quarter of people showing an improvement, a quarter showing a decline and around a half of people showing no change in this period (Thomas and Kerr, 2011).

In terms of design, the strongest study published at the time of writing is a large RCT of an 8-week programme of health promotion classes designed for adults with intellectual disabilities, with 443 participants and follow-up measurement one year after the intervention was completed (McDermott et al., 2012). This study found that participation in the health promotion classes did not have a significant impact on people's engagement in moderate to vigorous physical activity or their BMI one year after the completion of the intervention.

Several reasons have been posited for the findings from this body of research. Many of the programmes seem atheoretical, with no clear underpinning in theories of health behaviour change or consideration of how such theories may apply or need adapting for people with intellectual disabilities (Ravesloot et al., 2011). Many interventions also lack clarity in regard to the components of the programme, a clear rationale for the components included in the programme, or clarity about the intended outcomes of the programme, making the identification of effective components difficult (Seekins et al., 2010).

Perhaps most importantly, a number of authors have suggested that the effectiveness or otherwise of health promotion programmes for people with intellectual disabilities are massively influenced by the physical, social and economic environments within which they live (Heller et al., 2011; Marks, Sisirak, Heller and Wagner, 2010; McDermott et al., 2012; Thomas and Kerr, 2011). The supportiveness or otherwise of other people who play an important part in the daily lives of people with intellectual disabilities, such as family members or paid support staff, seem to have a major influence on the extent to which people with intellectual disabilities engage in any health promotion activities offered to them. Furthermore, for those people with intellectual disabilities living in residential service settings, the resources and routines of these residential settings can either help or hinder opportunities to engage in health promotion programmes. The relationship between health knowledge, health behaviours and health outcomes for people with intellectual disabilities is certainly far from straightforward (McDermott et al., 2012), providing further support for the contention that people with intellectual disabilities are often living in environments that impede self-determination when it comes to health matters (Blacher and Begum, 2011; Krahn and Campbell, 2011; Shogren et al., 2006).

A broader scoping review of 79 studies concerning the impact of health promotion programmes on the health of disabled people, from which the literature for the intellectual disability review was drawn (Heller et al., 2011), reported on health promotion programmes largely aimed at specific disability groups rather than pan-disability health promotion interventions (Seekins et al., 2010). Similar methodological limitations as those mentioned above were reported, such that no definitive conclusions about the effectiveness of such programmes could be drawn.

A Cochrane systematic review of interventions for promoting physical activity amongst adults in the general population (Foster et al., 2005) concluded that physical activity interventions have a moderate effect on self-reported physical activity, although they also reported huge variations in methodology and findings across studies. The review did not mention whether disabled people generally or people with intellectual disabilities in particular were included in the reviewed studies, although studies involving people living in institutions were excluded from the review.

In addition to the health-promotion research concerning nutrition, physical activity and/or weight loss for adults with intellectual disabilities, there is a smaller research literature concerning similar health promotion activities directed towards children and/or adolescents with intellectual disabilities. For example, pre–post evaluations (some with comparison groups) of exercise training for children or adolescents with intellectual disabilities have reported short-term improvements in weight, BMI and indicators of physical fitness (Elmahgoub et al., 2009; Golubovic, Maksimovic and Glumbic, 2012; Stanish and Temple, 2012). Less evidence appears to be available concerning programmes combining nutrition, physical activity and weight loss components (Fleming et al., 2008; Simpson et al., 2006).

Systematic reviews of research evidence concerning children and adolescents in the general population suggest that school-based interventions designed to promote physical activity and fitness in children and adolescents have a positive impact on the duration of physical activity, indicators of physical fitness and reduced time spent watching television, with combined educational materials and changes to school curricula the minimum required to achieve these improvements (Dobbins et al., 2009). Systematic reviews of interventions both to treat and prevent obesity in children conclude that multi-component interventions are most likely to be effective, although heterogeneity in intervention components and study design make definitive conclusions difficult (Luttikhuis et al., 2009; Waters et al., 2011). None of these systematic reviews mention disabled children, although studies could be excluded from the reviews if participants were children with 'severe co-morbidities' or reported conditions such as Prader–Willi Syndrome.

Smoking, alcohol misuse and illegal drug use

Some published research is available concerning health education/counselling programmes targeted at other types of health behaviour change amongst people with intellectual disabilities.

For example, despite variable and sometimes high rates of smoking reported amongst people with intellectual disabilities in specialist residential services (Steinberg, Heimlich and Williams, 2009), reports of the development and evaluation of smoking-cessation programmes with education and/or psychosocial components specifically for people with intellectual disabilities are sparse and mixed in their reported achievement of smoking cessation rather than smoking reduction (Singh et al., 2011; Sturmey, Lee and Robek, 2003; Tracy and Hosken, 1997). As with the literature concerning diet and physical activity reported above, residential environments can act to reinforce smoking behaviour and hinder the effectiveness of smoking-reduction programmes, for example by using cigarettes as a reinforcer in a token economy programme (Peine et al., 1998) or by residential staff smoking in the person's home (Sturmey et al., 2003).

In contrast, there is a substantial evidence base concerning the efficacy and effectiveness of smoking cessation education and counselling programmes for the general population (Killoran and Bauld, 2006; Lancaster and Stead, 2008; Stead and Lancaster, 2009). In terms of efficacy, both individual and group counselling have been found in systematic reviews to be efficacious in helping people to stop smoking, although the inclusion of people with intellectual disabilities in these studies is not reported (Lancaster and Stead, 2008; Stead and Lancaster, 2009). An evaluation of a national smoking cessation programme in the UK reported that it was successful in encouraging higher rates of access to smoking cessation by people from economically disadvantaged groups, although smoking cessation rates were lower amongst these groups (Killoran and Bauld, 2006). Disabled people were not a priority group for these smoking-cessation services (Pound et al., 2005), and the extent to which people with intellectual disabilities accessed and benefitted from these services was not reported, although one study has reported that general population smoking-cessation materials required extensive adaptation for people with intellectual disabilities in Australia (Tracy and Hosken, 1997).

Health education and counselling interventions to reduce alcohol and illegal drug misuse amongst people with intellectual disabilities are similarly sparsely reported (Chapman and Wu, 2012; McGillicuddy, 2006a). A randomised controlled trial (42 participants per study arm) of a 10-week substance education and skills-building programme for adults with intellectual disabilities reported that the programme improved participants' knowledge but did not change substance-related attitudes or behaviours (McGillicuddy and Blane, 1999). There is some evidence from the USA that between 2% and 3% of youths or adults with intellectual disabilities have received some form of substance use-related treatment, with people with intellectual disabilities less likely to initiate or engage in treatment and more likely to drop out of treatment than other groups (Larson, Lakin and Huang, 2003; Slayter, 2008, 2010a, 2010b). Furthermore, the engagement of people with intellectual disabilities in these types of treatment may be socially patterned, with non-White groups, people with serious mental health problems and people living in non-urban areas more likely to be coded as receiving substance use-related treatment (Slayter, 2010b).

Systematic reviews of educational and psychosocial interventions designed to reduce alcohol misuse in the general population have reported limited evidence for the effectiveness of Alcoholics Anonymous-style abstinence programmes (Ferri, Amato and Davoli, 2006), but some evidence for the effectiveness of brief counselling interventions in primary healthcare settings (Kaner et al., 2007). There is also some evidence for the effectiveness of school- and family-based psychosocial programmes designed to prevent the establishment of alcohol misuse amongst young people (Foxcroft and Tsertsvadze, 2011). There currently seems to be less conclusive evidence concerning the effectiveness of psychosocial interventions to reduce the misuse of illegal drugs amongst the general population (Denis et al., 2006; Knapp, Soares, Farrell and Silva de Lima, 2007; Mayet et al., 2005). In all these systematic reviews, whether people with intellectual disabilities were included and the relative effectiveness of programmes for people with intellectual disabilities are not reported.

Oral health

A small number of studies have evaluated health education programmes to improve the generally poor oral health of people with intellectual disabilities (Anders, 2010), typically directed to caregivers of people with intellectual disabilities. These studies have reported improvements in knowledge (either amongst people with intellectual disabilities or their caregivers) and oral hygiene behaviour, although these studies have typically used pre–post designs with no comparison groups (Faulks and Hennequin, 2000; Fickert and Ross, 2012). Reviews of health promotion and education concerning oral health with children, adolescents and adults in the general population have reported some overall improvements in oral hygiene behaviour but more transient impacts on knowledge and attitudes (Brown, 1994; Brukiene and Aleksejuniene J., 2009; Renz et al., 2007).

Sexual health

There are increasing calls for the human rights of people with intellectual disabilities to be recognised with respect to their sexuality and sexual behaviour (Tilley et al., 2012), and an increasing evidence base demonstrating suppression of both people's sexuality and sexual behaviour (particularly likely in specialist residential services), and potentially risky sexual behaviours (potentially more likely amongst adults with intellectual disabilities not known to specialist services) amongst people with intellectual disabilities (Servais, 2006). However, evaluations of sexual health education and/or promotion programmes are relatively sparse and methodologically limited, involving small samples for people with intellectual disabilities known to specialist services and almost always focusing exclusively on women. The largest body of literature concerns psycho-educational programmes for women with intellectual disabilities with the aim of helping them protect themselves from sexual violence (Doughty and Kane, 2010; Barger et al., 2009), which report short-term self-report changes but do not evaluate longer-term behavioural changes. There are also scattered, small-scale evaluations of other sexual health education/promotion programmes specifically for adults with intellectual disabilities, such as an HIV/AIDS knowledge programme for women (Wells et al., 2012), a programme to improve decision-making capacity concerning sex (Dukes and McGuire, 2009), programmes to improve knowledge and safe sexual behaviour concerning dating and relationships (Gardiner and Braddon, 2009; Ward et al., 2012) and a psycho-educational group for men who have sex with men (Withers et al., 2001).

A recent systematic review of the general population research reports that comprehensive group-based risk-reduction programmes with adolescents are effective in preventing or reducing the risk of adolescent pregnancy and sexually transmitted infections, although no conclusions could be drawn on the effectiveness of abstinence education programmes (Chin et al., 2012). Many of the interventions for people with intellectual disabilities described above are similar in their approach to risk-reduction programmes, although programmes with people with intellectual disabilities tend to focus on women rather than on both genders, and tend to occur in adulthood rather than adolescence, possibly due to some reluctance on the part of both parents and educators (Pownall et al., 2012; Wilkenfeld and Ballan, 2011).

Mental health

Although not typically considered as a health education or counselling intervention, psychotherapies to address mental health problems amongst people with intellectual disabilities (including behavioural, cognitive-behavioural and psychodynamic approaches) explicitly require informed consent and are psychosocial interventions designed to result in improvements in mental health. Although there has been a steady increase in evaluations of psychosocial interventions aimed at improving a wide range of mental health and psychological problems experienced by adults with intellectual disabilities, such as anxiety, depression, anger, interpersonal problems and psychosis, these are typically limited in terms of sample size and methodology (large-scale randomised controlled trials are very rare). Published findings tend to report some improvements in mental health amongst adults with intellectual disabilities known to specialist services, although it is difficult to conclude which components of these psychosocial interventions are effective, and both cognitive-behavioural and psychodynamic approaches can place substantial cognitive and linguistic demands on clients (Prout, 2003, 2011; Taylor et al., 2013).

In the UK, significant investment has gone into a national programme of psychological interventions for adults with common mental health problems, Improving Access to Psychological Therapies (IAPT) (www.iapt.nhs.uk). IAPT is based in primary healthcare settings and has ambitions to be easy to access and universal in its coverage, including being inclusive to people with intellectual disabilities (Department of Health, 2009). Approved IAPT interventions are drawn from evidence-based guidance for clinical practice developed by the National Institute for Health and Clinical Excellence (www.nice.org.uk). However, the research underpinning this clinical guidance derives from RCTs that often explicitly exclude people with intellectual disabilities, and within IAPT data collection systems and evaluations there has been no identification of people with intellectual disabilities or determination of the relative effectiveness of IAPT services for people with intellectual disabilities compared with other groups (Richards and Borglin, 2011; Taylor et al., 2013).

Summary

Taken together, these findings suggest that health education programmes aimed at individual health behaviour change amongst people with intellectual disabilities are likely to have a limited long-term impact in the absence of environments that consistently reinforce the messages and activities contained in these programmes. There are also issues around informed consent and meaningful participation in such programmes for a substantial sub-population of people with intellectual disabilities.

Furthermore, there is very little evidence concerning the effectiveness of health education and/or promotion programmes directed towards adults with intellectual disabilities not known to specialist intellectual disability services or people with intellectual disabilities in low- and middle-income countries, with programmes directed largely towards adults rather than children or adolescents, where the general population literature suggests they may be more effective.

Finally, health education/promotion programmes for the general population seem to operate either an explicit or a de facto exclusion policy with regard to people with intellectual disabilities. There is no evidence at present to make comparative judgements about health education/promotion programmes targeted specifically at people with intellectual disabilities versus programmes designed for whole populations and inclusive to people with intellectual disabilities.

Level 2: clinical interventions

Interventions at this level constitute the bulk of activity within health services, including surgical and drug treatments for existing acute and long-term health conditions. These may have protective functions for at-risk groups (for example, statins for control of cholesterol) but require ongoing intervention.

As this book is concerned with a public health perspective we will not be comprehensively reviewing the evidence concerning clinical interventions for specific health problems experienced by people with intellectual disabilities – other excellent overviews of clinical interventions are available (O'Hara, McCarthy and Bouras, 2010a). From a public health perspective, questions tend to centre on the health systems and services within which clinical interventions take place. Two major questions arise when taking such a public health perspective on clinical interventions for people with intellectual disabilities.

First, does the population of people with intellectual disabilities have access to the range of clinical interventions required for their health needs? Potential issues here concern whether health systems and health services can identify the population of people with intellectual disabilities and their likely profile of health problems requiring clinical interventions. A further issue here is whether health systems and health services either inadvertently or intentionally deny access to people with intellectual disabilities from needed clinical interventions, for example through inaccessible processes for making health service appointments.

Second, are clinical interventions equally effective for people with intellectual disabilities compared with other sub-groups of the general population? Across a range of clinical interventions, behaviour change in patients is crucial to the success of the intervention, ranging from postoperative recovery programmes through to ongoing adherence to medication regimens and the long-term management of chronic health conditions. Do people with intellectual disabilities engage effectively in these aspects of clinical interventions, and are health services set up to facilitate this?

In trying to address the first question, a major issue is the relative lack of visibility of people with intellectual disabilities within standard health system databases and public health surveillance systems, particularly adults with intellectual disabilities not using specialist intellectual disability services, as we discussed in Chapters 3 and 4 (Glover et al., 2011; Krahn et al., 2010).

As discussed earlier, the available evidence is inconsistent concerning the rates at which people with intellectual disabilities visit primary healthcare practitioners compared with the general population (Kerr, Richards and Glover, 1996; Whitfield, Langan and Russell, 1996; Turk et al., 2010), although as we have seen their health needs are likely to be greater and their rates of primary healthcare consultation are lower than would be expected when compared with groups with other long-term conditions (Felce et al., 2008b). Regarding secondary healthcare, there is some evidence that people with intellectual disabilities experience increased uptake of medical and dental hospital services but a reduced uptake of surgical specialities compared with the general population (Morgan, Ahmed and Kerr, 2000), a greater number of preventable hospitalisations (Balogh et al., 2005), greater use of emergency hospital services rather than hospital outpatient care amongst people with intellectual disabilities living in more deprived areas (Cooper et al., 2011), and a greater proportion of potentially preventable emergency hospital admissions compared with the general population (Glover and Evison, 2013).

These results, taken together with evidence of considerable unmet health needs amongst people with intellectual disabilities (Alborz, McNally and Glendinning, 2005; Beange, McElduff and Baker, 1995) and evidence that service usage does not map on to likely need for clinical interventions within the population of people with intellectual disabilities (Cooper, 1997a; Turk et al., 2010), strongly suggest that people with intellectual disabilities are not accessing health services proportionate to their health needs. 'Reasonable adjustments' developed by health systems and health services to improve the accessibility of health services to people with intellectual disabilities have not yet been rigorously evaluated (Hatton et al., 2011), with the exception of health checks (to be discussed as a Level 3 public health intervention below).

There is also limited evidence concerning the second question: whether clinical interventions are equally effective for people with intellectual disabilities compared with other sub-groups of the general population. There is some scattered evidence that people with intellectual disabilities can have poor experiences of clinical interventions (broadly defined), although comparisons to the experiences of the general population are lacking. Examples include:

- In the UK, there have been many documented examples of secondary health services causing the preventable death of people with intellectual disabilities, with contributory factors reported to include poor communication, a failure of health service staff to recognise pain, delays in diagnosis and treatment, a lack of basic care, and the use of Do Not Resuscitate orders (Heslop et al., 2013; Mencap, 2007; 2012a).
- Research concerning cancer services for people with intellectual disabilities reports that people with intellectual disabilities with cancer are less likely to be informed of their diagnosis and prognosis, be given pain relief, be involved in decisions about their care and receive palliative care (Bernal, 2008; Tuffrey-Wijne, Hogg and Curfs, 2007).

- Research consistently shows that a very high proportion of people with intellectual disabilities are receiving prescribed psychotropic medication, most commonly anti-psychotic medication (40–44% long-stay hospitals; 19–32% community-based residential homes; 9–10% family homes). Anti-psychotics are most commonly prescribed for challenging behaviours rather than psychosis, despite no evidence for their effectiveness in treating challenging behaviours and considerable evidence of harmful side effects (de Kuijper et al., 2010; Emerson and Einfeld, 2011; Molyneux, Emerson and Caine, 1999; Robertson et al., 2000a, 2005).
- Surgical interventions for congenital heart abnormalities have historically often been denied to children with Down's syndrome (who are at high risk of such congenital heart abnormalities) with no medical basis (Amark and Sunnegardh, 1999), although research suggests that the proportion of children with Down's syndrome and congenital heart abnormalities undergoing surgery is increasing, and their survival rate after surgery is also improving (Irving and Chaudhari, 2012).

In summary, health services for the general population seem to struggle to provide health interventions that are accessible and effective for people with intellectual disabilities. Furthermore, gaps in health surveillance systems make it difficult to identify and investigate these issues to provide comparative data on health intervention accessibility and effectiveness.

Level 3: long-lasting protective interventions

Interventions at this level are interventions that need to occur only once or infrequently, with the aim of protecting individuals against the onset of health problems. Typical interventions at this level include vaccination programmes and health screening programmes, although they do require the participation and consent of individuals. Most of this section will focus on health screening programmes, but at the end of the section we will outline a very different type of long-lasting protective intervention, the provision of local area-based interventions for disadvantaged families with young children designed to improve the health and well-being of children, such as Head Start in the USA and Sure Start in the UK (Melhuish et al., 2010).

The biggest evidence base for long-lasting protective interventions for people with intellectual disabilities concerns health screening and regular, preventive health checks. Unlike other parts of this chapter, we will outline the evidence concerning the access of people with intellectual disabilities to general population screening programmes before we outline the evidence concerning health checks designed specifically for people with intellectual disabilities. This is because health checks specifically designed for people with intellectual disabilities are in part a policy response to the poor access to general population screening programmes experienced by people with intellectual disabilities.

Although evidence is patchy, there is consistent evidence that people with intellectual disabilities and their family carers are less likely than non-disabled people to be supported to access a range of general population health screening programmes, resulting in poorer access to a range of health screening programmes, including:

- routine dental check-ups (Barr et al., 1999; Emerson et al., 2005; Havercamp et al., 2004; Owens et al., 2010);
- routine check-ups/screening for vision or hearing impairments (McGlade et al., 2010; Lavis, Cullen and Roy, 1997; Yeates, 1995);
- cervical smear screening (Havercamp et al., 2004; Djuretic et al., 1999; Osborn et al., 2012; Parish et al., 2006; Pearson et al., 1998; Reynolds, Stanistreet and Elton, 2008), although certain sub-groups of women with intellectual disabilities (e.g. women aged over 35 years) may show higher rates of access to screening compared with their general-population peers (Lin et al., 2010b);
- colonoscopy and colorectal cancer screening (Fischer et al., 2012; Osborn et al., 2012);
- breast self-examination and mammography (Havercamp et al., 2004; Davies and Duff, 2001; Djuretic et al., 1999; Osborn et al., 2012; Parish et al., 2006; Swaine et al., 2013; Truesdale-Kennedy et al., 2011; Piachaud and Rohde, 1998; Willis et al,. 2008);
- testicular self-examination and prostate cancer screening (Osborn et al., 2012; Peate and Maloret, 2007).

UK evidence suggests no systematic improvements in the rates of people with intellectual disabilities accessing a range of general-population cancer screening programmes (Osborn et al., 2012), while US evidence suggests that adults with intellectual disabilities living with families are less likely than those living in residential settings to receive a range of preventive healthcare interventions (Bershadsky et al., 2012).

There is very little research evidence concerning vaccination rates for people with intellectual disabilities compared with the general population. Research in Taiwan reports lower rates of influenza and hepatitis B vaccination coverage amongst children and adolescents with intellectual disabilities (Lin et al., 2010a; Yen et al., 2012), but a US study reports higher rates of influenza vaccination amongst working-age women with intellectual disabilities living in community settings (Parish et al., 2006). Young children with cognitive delays in Bangladesh, Laos and Mongolia (but not Thailand) have been reported to be less likely to receive BCG, polio, diphtheria and measles/MMR vaccinations than children without cognitive delay (Llewellyn et al., 2012).

In summary, the evidence suggests that people with intellectual disabilities are substantially less likely to access a broad range of mainstream health screening programmes. The barriers to access reported for access to health services generally (discussed above) also apply with regard to accessing health screening. As with the other evidence reviewed in this chapter, the evidence here is largely restricted to high-income countries, and to those adults with intellectual disabilities who are recognised as such within healthcare databases.

Partly as a response to the evidence concerning poor access to mainstream health screening programmes, some countries such as England have financially incentivised primary care general health practitioners to provide regular (usually annual) health checks specifically for adults with intellectual disabilities.

In terms of coverage, after four years of the financial incentives being offered to general practitioners in England, just over half of eligible adults with intellectual disabilities (53%, or 82,777 people) were reported as receiving a health check in 2011/12, up from 23% in 2008/9. There was also substantial variation in coverage between local health boards (called at the time Primary Care Trusts (PCTs) in England); in 2011/12 the bottom 10% of PCTs reported 28% of eligible adults with intellectual disabilities receiving an annual health check compared with 73% of eligible adults in the top 10% of PCTs (Glover et al., 2012b, 2013).

A recent mixed-method study of health checks in England suggests a number of possible facilitators and barriers to the widespread uptake of effective health checks for people with intellectual disabilities. Facilitators included general practitioners perceiving that there was a value to health checks over and above routine primary care practice; the continued financial incentive for conducting health checks (suggesting that such health checks are not becoming embedded within routine primary care practice); clarity about how many people with intellectual disabilities are eligible (which relies on robust data systems for flagging people with intellectual disabilities); general practitioner confidence in their skills in working with people with intellectual disabilities; and clear leadership from health service commissioners (Chauhan et al., 2012; Turner and Robinson, 2010).

A recent systematic review has summarised the evidence concerning the impact of health checks for people with intellectual disabilities (Robertson et al., 2011), including three randomised controlled trials (Jones and Kerr, 1997; Lennox et al., 2007, 2010), a cohort study (Cooper et al., 2006) and a study systematically varying the length of interval between repeated health checks (Felce et al., 2008a).

Across the research literature, before receiving health checks between 51% and 94% of people with intellectual disabilities had previously undetected health conditions (Baxter et al., 2006; Cassidy et al., 2002), and the health checks detected between 2.2 and 5.2 additional diagnoses (Carlsen and Galluzzi, 1994; Hahn and Aronow, 2005). A pooled analysis of three studies with control groups reported substantially increased (odds ratio ≥1.5, although most of these increases did not reach statistical significance due to wide confidence intervals) identification of psychiatric disorder, heart disease, reflux disease, hypertension, constipation and 'other' diseases (Lennox et al., 2011). In addition to these 'major' health conditions, other 'minor' health conditions (which can have a major impact on the person's combined capabilities) are commonly reported, such as ear wax (with concomitant temporary hearing impairment), skin problems, dental problems, constipation, anaemia and foot problems (Robertson et al., 2011). Additional unmet health needs continue to be identified in repeated health checks, with no association between the number of additional unmet health needs identified and the length of time between health checks (Felce et al., 2008a).

In addition to increased detection of previously unrecognised minor and major health conditions, there is also consistent evidence that health checks lead to targeted actions to address the health needs identified in the health check (Robertson et al., 2011), with the pooled analysis suggesting large (odds ratio ≥3.8) and statistically significant increases in vision and hearing testing, and hepatitis B and tetanus/diphtheria vaccination compared with control groups (Lennox et al., 2011). However, a recent UK study suggests that follow-up health screening/interventions after a health check are weighted towards health conditions that are also financially incentivised for general practitioners, with less attention paid to health issues such as sensory impairments or mental health problems that are particularly pertinent to the population of people with intellectual disabilities (Chauhan et al., 2012).

Compared with the evidence on the impact of health checks on the detection of unmet health needs and on subsequent health service activity, there is very little research concerning the impact of health checks on the health of people with intellectual disabilities. The available evidence tends to come from studies that are less strong methodologically, but they do report a range of short-term health gains potentially attributable to health checks (Robertson et al., 2011).

In summary, regular health checks for people with intellectual disabilities seem to be effective in detecting the unmet health needs of such people and in triggering further health screening/assessment, health intervention and health advice. There is currently little methodologically compelling evidence concerning the medium- or long-term impact of regular health checks on the health of people with intellectual disabilities. There do, however, seem to be substantial barriers to the routine implementation of health checks for people with intellectual disabilities within mainstream primary care health services. Finally, it is important to note that the majority of adults with mild/moderate intellectual disabilities will not be flagged as such in general practice databases and, even if they were flagged, would not be eligible for financially incentivised annual health checks as they are currently implemented.

As mentioned at the start of the section, we will conclude this section by outlining the evidence concerning local area-based services for disadvantaged families with young children, which have the explicit aim of improving children's long-term prospects in terms of health, well-being and educational attainment. Evidence from US and UK studies suggests that such initiatives can have substantial medium-term positive impacts on children and families, including children and families in the most disadvantaged circumstances which are likely to include substantial numbers of children at risk of becoming classified as having an intellectual disability (Melhuish, Belsky and Barnes, 2010), although results are rarely reported in ways that children with intellectual disabilities can be identified (Emerson et al., 2011d). The intervention with the most substantial evidence base concerns a version of the Triple-P behavioural family intervention designed for children with disabilities, called Stepping Stones Triple-P. Triple-P operates on an area basis, with five levels of intervention of increasing intensity designed to identify families needing any level of intervention in the area and offer the minimum level of intervention required to meet the needs of individual families. A recent systematic review of 12 studies concerning Stepping Stones Triple-P on families with a child with disabilities (the nature of the disability varied across studies, but largely focused on children with intellectual and/or developmental disabilities) reported statistically significant, moderate to large improvements in child behaviour problems, and parenting styles, satisfaction, efficacy and relationship (Tellegen and Sanders, 2013). However, no analysis was possible of the impact of these programmes on inequalities within the population of families with a child with disabilities, or on the differential impact of Stepping Stones Triple-P versus Triple-P for general-population families.

Area-based urban regeneration/public health initiatives designed to improve the economies and health of deprived communities in the UK focused more on adults (Cummins, 2010), have been systematically reviewed in terms of their potential impact on population health (Thomson et al., 2006). Although methodologies varied and results were mixed, there was some evidence for positive impacts on population health in these areas. Evaluation of an area-based initiative more focused on health in deprived communities, the New Deal for Communities programme, has reported minor (and not statistically significant) improvements in psychological well-being, smoking cessation, consumption of fruit and vegetables and limiting long-term illness, although the degree to which these are specifically associated with New Deal for Communities areas is unclear (Stafford et al., 2008). Again, the impact of these area-based programmes on people with intellectual disabilities is not reported, and the extent to which such area-based programmes reach and positively impact upon the population of people with intellectual disabilities is currently unclear.

Level 4: changing the context to make individuals' default decisions healthy

The two layers at the base of the pyramid are qualitatively different from the three layers of the pyramid discussed so far, in that they intervene at the level of people's environments and do not require active participation and consent from individuals at all.

Public health interventions at this level aim to change the environmental contexts within which people live to ensure that healthy options are the default options, such that people would have to make active efforts not to benefit from them. Examples of public health interventions at this level would include fluoridation of the water supply, measures to reduce air and water pollution, banning smoking in public places, placing high levels of tax on unhealthy foods and designing communities to enhance the safety of physical activities such as walking and cycling.

Although the vast majority of public health interventions at this level are designed to influence the health of the general population, there are some examples of interventions of this type designed specifically to improve the health of people with intellectual disabilities. These typically involve the sub-population of people with intellectual disabilities who spend most of their lives in specialist intellectual disability service environments, particularly residential services of various types. Given that this group of people with intellectual disabilities spend so much of their time in service environments, the lack of evidence on designing service structures and practices to make people's default decisions healthy is surprising.

One obvious area where intellectual disability services could intervene to make people's default decisions healthy concerns nutrition. A recent systematic review of the evidence concerning nutrition and adults with intellectual disabilities documented the poor nutritional status of adults with intellectual disabilities across a range of residential settings, despite methodological difficulties in establishing nutritional status in this group (Humphries, Traci and Seekins, 2009b). The review also suggested that service practices play an important role in promoting (or not) healthy nutrition amongst residents, particularly in terms of the range of foods offered from which choices could be made and in the nutrition support offered to more independent residents (Humphries et al., 2009b). Evidence is sparse on the effectiveness of nutrition support interventions in residential settings, but evidence from one study focusing on supporting staff to improve the nutritional adequacy of menus (including support in terms of meal planning, shopping, cooking) in group homes reported an improvement in the nutritional adequacy of food menus (although changes in the health status of residents were not assessed) (Humphries et al., 2009a; Stafford et al., 2008).

Other similar public health interventions specifically designed to operate within intellectual disability services, such as smoking bans, have not been systematically evaluated.

Of potentially greater importance for the entire population of people with intellectual disabilities are public health interventions designed to make the default decisions of the entire population healthier, such as smoking bans in public places. Evaluating the health impact of such interventions is methodologically complex, and policy interventions are rarely based on robust evidence (Law, 2010).

Evaluating the specific health impact of such interventions on the population is further complicated by the environments within which people with intellectual disabilities live and spend their time. For example, people with intellectual disabilities in some forms of residential service or day service will be spending much of their time in segregated, semi-public environments with a continuous staff presence, with workplace health and safety restrictions applying that would not apply in the homes of the general population. People in such restricted environments may also spend relatively little time in local community environments, with relatively little contact with other people in local communities and little engagement with community facilities or activities. They may also have relatively little disposable income and have little control over access to food, alcohol, cigarettes or other items with an impact on health. People with intellectual disabilities not in contact with specialist intellectual disability services are much more likely to be similar to the general population living in deprived communities, where there are consistent concerns that general public health interventions may have comparatively little impact (Graham and Power, 2010).

Some examples of general-population public-health interventions designed to make individuals' default decisions healthy will be presented here, to illustrate their potential for improving the health of people with intellectual disabilities and also the complexities of their application to people with intellectual disabilities.

One example where there is evidence of general population health impact concerns smoking bans in public places, which have been adopted in several US states and high-income countries around the world. Workplace smoking bans have been reported to have short-term impacts both on smokers' attempts to quit and the success rates of their quit attempts (Heloma et al., 2001). Workplace smoking bans are less likely to have an impact on the population of smokers with intellectual disabilities, as they are less likely to be present in workplaces (either in residential settings or unemployed). They may, however, have a positive impact on passive smoking by reducing staff smoking where residential and day services are treated as workplaces, although research from psychiatric inpatient settings suggests that smoking bans without the force of legislation are limited in their impact (Lawn and Pols, 2005). A systematic review of legislatively enforced smoking bans in public places suggests a positive impact of smoking bans on improved cardiovascular health, with the positive impact increasing in accordance with the length of time the ban has been enforced (Meyers, Neuberger and He, 2009). A positive impact on people with intellectual disabilities will be largely dependent on the extent to which they spend time in those public places affected by smoking bans, which is likely to be considerably reduced for those people with intellectual disabilities receiving intellectual disability services.

Another public health intervention relating to smoking concerns increasing taxation on tobacco products. General population evidence suggests that increasing the price of tobacco through taxation has a positive impact on decisions to quit taken by smokers, with a potentially bigger impact on people from lower socio-economic groups (Ludbrook, 2010). This would suggest a potentially positive impact on people with intellectual disabilities not in contact with specialist intellectual disability services.

Another class of public health interventions concerns modifying people's environments to increase the likelihood of them engaging in more physical activity, particularly walking and cycling. Government-sponsored reviews of this class of public health intervention have recently been conducted in the UK and the USA, summarised and synthesised in Crombie, Killoran and Naidoo (2010) and Gebel, Bauman and Bull (2010). Evaluating such interventions is methodologically complex, and few studies directly evaluating the impact of environmental changes have been published to date. For the general population, the sparse evidence suggests that:

- Traffic-calming measures in urban environments can result in small increases in walking and cycling.
- The development of walking/cycling trails can result in increased walking and cycling activity, although these increases may be largely amongst people who are already physically active.
- Urban initiatives to discourage car use, such as road closures in Bogota or the introduction of the congestion charge in London, can result in increases in walking and cycling to work and increased use of public transport.
- Increasing the density of urban public transport stops can lead to increases in the use of public transport to work and small increases in walking to public transport stops.
- Evidence concerning the impact of other urban micro-environmental initiatives, such as improving street lighting or increasing the 'walkability' of urban environments, on physical activity is lacking.

Again, evidence concerning the impact of such environmental public health initiatives on the population of people with intellectual disabilities is lacking. It is possible that many of these initiatives will have relatively little impact on people with intellectual disabilities, as they are less likely to be engaged in regular commuting journeys to urban workplaces, possibly less likely to be cycle owners who are proficient in cycling, and less likely to find public transport accessible.

In summary, both within and beyond specialist intellectual disability services, there are multiple potential methods for designing the environments of people with intellectual disabilities in ways to promote healthy behaviours as the default option. However, such interventions within intellectual disability services have rarely been systematically evaluated, and general-population environmental interventions have rarely been considered or evaluated in terms of their likely relevance to and impact upon the health of people with intellectual disabilities.

Level 5: socio-economic factors

As we have seen, social and economic factors are substantial determinants of the health of people with intellectual disabilities (as they are for the rest of the population). Actions at this level aim to improve the social and economic conditions of populations or sub-populations with the ultimate aim of improving population health. Examples of such actions include poverty-reduction strategies, strategies to improve employment opportunities and, for disabled people, strategies to reduce stigma, discrimination and disablism throughout society. Clear linkages between actions at this level and improvements in population health can be difficult to establish, not least because whilst such actions may act to reduce health problems associated with poverty and associated early mortality, they may also act to increase health problems associated with affluence and increased longevity.

A relatively recent review of systematic reviews of interventions designed to tackle the wider social determinants of health inequalities in the general populations of high-income countries (Bambra et al., 2010) focused on the evidence concerning interventions designed to improve housing and living environments, improve work environments, improve transport and access to services, and address unemployment and welfare, agriculture and food, and water and sanitation. In general, the evidence base in each area was too heterogeneous to draw firm conclusions from the available evidence. However, there were some suggestions concerning the potential impact of such socio-economic interventions, such as:

- Rent assistance and other measures to improve housing mobility and choice for low-income families were associated with small improvements in self-reported general health and mental health.
- Improvements in housing quality (particularly related to keeping homes warm) were associated with improvements in self-reported health, particularly for groups with particular health problems (Thomson et al., 2013).
- Environmental changes designed to reduce the risks of falls (or injuries generally) resulted in reductions in the number of falls (but not injuries generally).
- Interventions in work environments designed to increase employee control in their jobs resulted in consistently positive effects on employee health, particularly mental health.

Few of the systematic reviews cited (or the studies included within them) investigated the impact of such interventions on health inequalities, and disability was not cited as a relevant factor in the review of reviews. Large-scale anti-stigma campaigns concerning mental health have also been implemented in several countries with the aim of reducing general population stigma and improving help-seeking amongst people with mental health problems. Although methodological issues again hamper evaluation of the effectiveness of these campaigns, it does seem that they can reduce stigmatising attitudes amongst the general population, although knowledge of mental health issues and treatments, positive attitudes towards mental health issues and non-discriminatory health service staff may be more relevant factors in promoting help-seeking amongst people with mental health problems (Henderson, Evans-Lacko and Thornicroft, 2013).

Although associations between socio-economic inequalities and health have been clearly established (Wilkinson and Pickett, 2009), there is some debate about whether reduced economic inequalities associated with certain national welfare systems have yielded the expected degree of reduced health inequalities (Mackenbach, 2012; Popham, Dibben and Bambra, 2013). Proposed reasons for persistent health inequalities even in countries with welfare states designed to reduce socio-economic inequalities are all particularly pertinent to the population of people with intellectual disabilities compared with the rest of the population (Mackenbach, 2012):

(1) Inequalities in access to material and immaterial resources have not been eliminated by the welfare state, and are still substantial; (2) due to greater intergenerational mobility, the composition of lower socio-economic groups has become more homogeneous with regard to personal character-istics associated with ill-health; and (3) due to a change in epidemiologi-cal regime, in which consumption behaviour became the most important determinant of ill-health, the marginal benefits of the immaterial resources to which a higher social position gives access has increased. (Mackenbach, 2012, p. 761)

Conclusions

This chapter demonstrates the broad range of interventions with the potential to improve the health of people with intellectual disabilities and reduce the health inequalities experienced by this population. However, the available evidence suggests some paradoxes when interventions are considered through the prism of the public health pyramid.

First, the bulk of the evidence concerns levels 1 and 2 health interventions (counselling and education; clinical interventions) directed specifically towards adults with intellectual disabilities known to specialist services. However, such interventions, with their frequent reliance on active individual behaviour change and informed consent, may be relatively ineffective for those adults with intellectual disabilities known to specialist services who are less likely to be able to provide informed consent and who live in relatively restrictive and unhelpful (in terms of health) service environments. Such interventions also do not target the majority of adults with intellectual disabilities who will not be known to specialist intellectual disability services, and do not target children with intellectual disabilities. Furthermore, people with intellectual disabilities tend to be either explicitly or de facto excluded from or invisible within general-population health initiatives, such that reasonable adjustments are not considered or adopted and inequalities in access or impact are not evaluated.

With the exception of regular health checks for the sub-group of people with intellectual disabilities who are eligible for them, there is relatively little evi-dence concerning the design and impact of long-lasting protective interventions, although once again people with intellectual disabilities are likely to be excluded from many mainstream health interventions. Apart from regular health checks for adults, the most promising interventions are likely to be area-based early interven-tion preventive services for families with young children that are accessible and receptive to families with a young child at risk of intellectual disability. However, specific evidence concerning the impact on these interventions on children at risk of intellectual disability is lacking.

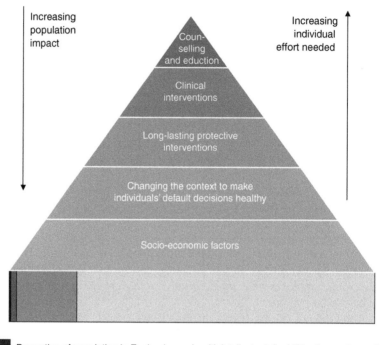

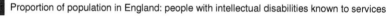

Figure 5.1 The health impact pyramid (adapted with permission from Frieden, 2010)

At the lower levels of the health impact pyramid, evidence concerning interventions that are likely to have the most substantial health impact on entire populations is lacking. These could be particularly relevant to the population of people
with intellectual disabilities, as they do not require informed consent and are
designed to make healthy options the easiest, default option. They would, however, require careful design and targeting to ensure that people with intellectual
disabilities were included. Interventions such as smoking bans, fiscal policies to
raise the prices of unhealthy goods, the redesign of urban environments, employment strategies and poverty reduction initiatives have not been considered in
terms of their relevance to or impact on the public health of people with intellectual disabilities.

Taken together, the available evidence suggests that a substantial shift is
required in our public health efforts for people with intellectual disabilities. Such
public health initiatives should look more towards designing 'healthy default'

environments rather than solely focusing on trying to achieve active individual behaviour change, should focus more on children at risk of intellectual disability, and should pay due attention to people with intellectual disabilities not known to specialist intellectual disability services.

6

Conclusions

Our aim in writing this book was to apply a public health lens (and more specifically a health inequalities lens) to further our understanding of the health of people with intellectual disabilities. We began the book by arguing that intellectual disability is an unavoidably social construct. We then outlined the capabilities framework (Nussbaum, 2009, 2011; Sen, 2001) and hopefully illustrated its potential utility for understanding both intellectual disability itself and the objectives of policies aiming to improve the health of people with intellectual disabilities. Throughout these discussions we demonstrated the importance of including social, economic and environment factors in any understanding of the development of intellectual disabilities.

In Chapter 2 we defined what is meant by health and briefly discussed how the health of groups or populations is typically measured. Following this, we discussed what is meant by the term health inequalities, and illustrated the extent of the health inequalities that occur between and within countries. We ended the chapter by summarising what is known about the causes of health inequalities in the general population. Whilst these determinants are undoubtedly complex, current knowledge highlights the importance of the 'social determinants' of health in driving the extensive differences in health status that have been repeatedly documented globally, regionally and within nations (World Health Organization, 2008; World Health Organization Regional Office for Europe, 2012).

In Chapter 3 we summarised what the available research literature tells us about the health status and needs of children and adults with intellectual disabilities. Given the availability of previous reviews, we focused on the 'big picture' and on more recent evidence as it relates to broad indicators of health (e.g. overall mortality, self-rated health) and specific health conditions and impairments. Notwithstanding the limitations of this evidence base, it is clear that in many, but not all, aspects of health, people with intellectual disabilities are disadvantaged when compared with their peers. In some areas (e.g. mortality, mental health, speech and communication disorders) these differences are stark. We need to keep in mind, however, that this body of evidence primarily relates to the 'visible minority' of people with more severe intellectual disabilities who are known to specialised intellectual disability services. We know much less about the health of the 'hidden majority' of people with mild intellectual disabilities, most of whom (as adults) are not known to specialised intellectual disability services.

In Chapter 4 we used Dahlgren and Whitehead's 'rainbow model' of the determinants of health (and health inequalities) (Dahlgren and Whitehead, 1991/2007) to better understand the health inequalities faced by people with intellectual disabilities. It is clear that people with intellectual disabilities are disadvantaged at every layer of this model. In Gloria Krahn's terms, they are subject to a cascade of disparities (Krahn and Fox, in press; Krahn, Hammond and Turner, 2006). Given the multiple and overlapping disadvantages faced by people with intellectual disabilities it is no surprise that they experience poorer health than their non-disabled peers. The available evidence also suggests that ameliorating the health inequalities faced by people with intellectual disabilities will require action at different levels of the determinants of the health 'rainbow'.

In Chapter 5 we reviewed what we know about the impact of a broad range of interventions on the health of people with intellectual disabilities and their capacity to reduce the health inequalities experienced by this population. We drew attention to the paradoxes that become evident when interventions are considered through the prism of the public health pyramid (Frieden, 2010). First, the bulk of the evidence concerns levels 1 and 2 health interventions (counselling and education; clinical interventions) directed specifically towards adults with intellectual disabilities known to specialist services. However, such interventions, with their frequent reliance on active individual behaviour change and informed consent, may be relatively ineffective for those adults with intellectual disabilities known to specialist services who are less likely to be able to provide informed consent and who live in relatively restrictive and unhelpful (in terms of health) service environments. Such interventions also do not target the majority of adults with intellectual disabilities who will not be known to specialist intellectual disability services, and do not target children with intellectual disabilities. Furthermore, people with intellectual disabilities (particularly those in the 'hidden majority') tend to be either explicitly or de facto excluded from or invisible within general-population health initiatives.

With the exception of regular health checks for people with intellectual disabilities, there is relatively little evidence concerning the design and impact of long-lasting protective interventions, although once again people with intellectual disabilities are likely to be excluded from many mainstream health interventions. Apart from regular health checks for adults, the most promising interventions are likely to be area-based early intervention preventive services for families with young children that are accessible and receptive to families with a young child at risk of intellectual disability. However, specific evidence concerning the impact on these interventions on children at risk of intellectual disability is lacking.

At the lowest levels of the health impact pyramid, evidence concerning interventions that are likely to have the most substantial health impact on the wider population of people with intellectual disabilities is lacking. Interventions such as smoking bans, fiscal policies to raise the prices of unhealthy goods, the redesign of urban environments, employment strategies and poverty-reduction initiatives have not been considered in terms of their relevance to or impact on the public health of people with intellectual disabilities.

Taken together, the available evidence suggests that a substantial shift is required in our public health efforts for people with intellectual disabilities. Such public health initiatives should look more towards designing 'healthy default' environments rather than solely focusing on trying to achieve active individual behaviour change, should focus more on children at risk of intellectual disability, and should pay due attention to people with intellectual disabilities not known to specialist intellectual disability services.

Challenges ahead

Viewing the health of people with intellectual disabilities through a public health lens, as we have tried to do throughout this book, has brought into sharp focus the broad array of challenges ahead if we are serious about improving the health of, and reducing the health inequalities experienced by, the whole population of people with intellectual disabilities. Although improving access to proactive and responsive health services is part of the equation, a public health approach requires a reach far beyond health services and far beyond the population of people with intellectual disabilities who are recognised as such within health and social care services. This final section of the book focuses on two areas where we think progress can (and needs to) be made: building a relevant knowledge base and changing policy and practice.

Building a relevant knowledge base

Writing this book was possible only because the quantity, quality and international reach of research and knowledge relevant to the public health of people with intellectual disabilities have rapidly improved over the past 20 years. However, this book also illustrates that, compared with public health research on the general population, we have a long way to go in generating comprehensive evidence concerning the public health of the entire population of people with intellectual disabilities, and generating evidence of the effectiveness (or otherwise) of public health interventions designed to improve the health of people with intellectual disabilities and reduce health inequalities between such people and the rest of the general population. We believe priorities for improved evidence would include (but would not be confined to) the following seven areas.

(1) **Adopting a life course perspective.** Life course perspectives dominate research on the determinants of health inequalities in the general population (Bartley, 2004; Davey Smith, 2002; Graham, 2007; Marmot and Wilkinson,

2006), and have drawn attention to the significance of early experience in shaping children's developmental health and their life trajectories (Irwin, Siddiqi and Hertzman, 2007). In contrast, the vast majority of research on the health of people with intellectual disabilities that we have discussed in the previous chapters has involved snapshots in time of the health of the 'visible minority' of adults with (more severe) intellectual disability who use intellectual disability services. We know remarkably little about the physical health of children with intellectual disability. What we do know, however, suggests that the health inequalities experienced by people with intellectual disabilities start early in life (see Table 3.2). For example, in both the UK and Australia children with intellectual disability show elevated rates of obesity by the time they enter school (Emerson, 2009; Emerson and Robertson, 2010). There is a pressing need for more longitudinal research on intellectual disability generally, and specifically in furthering our understanding the determinants of health inequalities experienced by people with intellectual disabilities. Using data already collected in large-scale longitudinal child development studies can provide a low-cost and highly efficient entry into the world of life course and longitudinal research (Emerson, 2012c).

(2) **Improving our understanding of the health of the 'hidden majority' of adults with mild intellectual disabilities**, who are not identified as such within health and social care services (Tymchuk, Lakin and Luckasson, 2001). For obvious reasons there are substantial methodological challenges here. One set of potential strategies involves linking the improved identification of children with mild intellectual disabilities in childhood to relevant data concerning the health of adults. This might include:

- Specialist longitudinal registers of the population of people with intellectual disabilities that continue to track all children with intellectual disabilities (including mild intellectual disabilities) through to adulthood within a geographically defined area.
- Using nationally representative birth cohort or other longitudinal cohort studies beginning in childhood to identify sub-populations of children with intellectual disabilities and tracking their health as adults.
- Conducting population-based surveys of adults with intellectual disabilities that include the identification of adults with mild intellectual disabilities.
- Linking databases identifying children with intellectual disabilities (e.g. within school systems) to general-population health databases (e.g. general practitioner databases).
- Developing short screening tools for use in general health service populations (e.g. primary care) to provide preliminary identifications of the potential population of adults with mild intellectual disabilities.

A second set of potential strategies for improving our knowledge of the health of the 'hidden majority' of adults with intellectual disabilities may involve adopting a health literacy lens rather than an intellectual disability lens. There is a substantial research literature reporting that a large proportion of the general adult population have limited health literacy. For example, systematic reviews of US studies have reported estimates of 26% of the adult US population with low literacy and a further 20% with marginal health literacy (Paasche-Orlow et al., 2005), systematic associations between poor child and parent health literacy and poorer child health outcomes (DeWalt and Hink, 2009; Sanders et al., 2009), but less evidence concerning the impact of interventions to improve health literacy (DeWalt and Hink, 2009; Sanders et al., 2009). Adults with mild intellectual disabilities should be part of the population with low or marginal health literacy (certainly education is robustly associated with health literacy), and connecting adults with intellectual disabilities to this research literature as a particularly high-risk population for low health literacy has the potential to generate substantial knowledge about the health needs and effectiveness of health services for this group.

(3) **Improving our understanding of the impact of social determinants on the health of people with more severe disabilities and on people with specific syndromes** associated with intellectual disability, such as autistic spectrum disorder. Because socio-economic gradients associated with the prevalence of severe intellectual disabilities and autism are less pronounced or even quite different to those for the prevalence of mild intellectual disabilities, there is a danger that the health of people with severe intellectual disabilities or associated syndromes is assumed to exist in a diagnostically overshadowed, biological/health service space existing outside the realm of social determinants. We need to understand which social determinants operate for these groups, particularly when people are living their lives in contexts substantially determined by service structures. This will mean a reappraisal of which social determinants are likely to have the greatest impact and how they can be assessed.

(4) **Understanding the impact of 'personal' discrimination on health.** In Chapter 4 we argued that, as with other marginalised or 'vulnerable' groups, exposure to overt acts of discrimination and violence is likely to be damaging to a person's health (Hughes et al., 2012; Krieger, 1999). We drew attention to the remarkably sparse literature on the exposure of people with intellectual disabilities to bullying, harassment, violence and abuse (Emerson and Roulstone, in press; Emerson et al., 2011a; Harrell, 2012; Murray and Powell, 2008; Sequeira and Hollins, 2003), but failed to find any population-based studies that drew connections between exposure to overt acts of discrimination and health. Filling this gap in our knowledge deserves some serious attention.

(5) **Improving our methods for estimating the entire population of people with intellectual disabilities, projecting population trends over time and modelling the impact of these trends on the health needs of this population.** Throughout this book we have seen the difficulties in generating estimates of the current population of people with intellectual disabilities and in trying to project population trends over time (Emerson and Hatton, 2011). We have also seen that the population of people with intellectual disabilities is potentially changing quite rapidly in public health terms, for example in increased

survival rates of people with more complex needs into adulthood, generally increasing life expectancy and potential changes in the ethnic composition of the population of people with intellectual disabilities in some high-income countries. Although more assumptions than are desirable are needed to produce such population estimates and projections, they are a necessary foundation for modelling the future public health needs of the population of people with intellectual disabilities.

(6) **Improving our understanding of which 'reasonable adjustments' work and why.** Recommendations for improving access to and the effectiveness of health services for people with intellectual disabilities are frequently framed in terms of health services making 'reasonable adjustments' or 'accommodations' to their practices, and there are numerous examples of such 'reasonable adjustments' being made within health services (Hatton et al., 2011) (or not) and of other reasonable adjustments, such as easy-read health information, changes to appointments procedures or the employment of specialist nurses within mainstream hospital services. Rigorous research is needed to evaluate both the effectiveness of such reasonable adjustments and how effective reasonable adjustments can be scaled up to become routine practice.

(7) **Improving the visibility of people with intellectual disabilities within mainstream public health research.** Much of the most ambitious public health research has evaluated large-scale interventions at national or multiple-area levels, which have been designed to alter the social determinants of health amongst entire communities (Killoran and Kelly, 2010). However, disability generally and people with intellectual disabilities in particular are invisible within such large-scale evaluations, as they are within large-scale evaluations of other public health interventions such as smoking cessation or weight loss interventions. In countries such as the UK, public health programmes that do not attempt to make reasonable adjustments and do not evaluate their relative impact on disabled people may not be compliant with legislation such as the Equality Act. In any event, the large numbers of people (including people with intellectual disabilities, other groups with cognitive impairments and people with low health literacy) who could potentially benefit from 'reasonably adjusted' public health interventions make a powerful argument that all public health interventions should be routinely 'reasonably adjusted'. Similarly, evaluations of such interventions should be similarly 'reasonably adjusted', such that people with intellectual disabilities can be identified within bigger population samples, the research methods and procedures are accessible to people with intellectual disabilities and/or proxy respondents, and the differential impact of public health interventions on people with intellectual disabilities can be analysed.

Changing policy and practice

In a recent review, Gloria Krahn and Michael Fox quoted Sir Charles Geoffrey Vickers, who in 1958 wrote, 'The landmarks of political, economic and social history are the moment when some condition passed from the category of the given into the category of the intolerable. I believe that the history of public health might well be written as a record of successive re-defining of the unacceptable'. They went on (perhaps somewhat optimistically) to argue that, 'we are in the midst of just such a time of re-definition … from accepting the poor health of people with intellectual disabilities as a given, to regarding these health disparities as intolerable' (Krahn and Fox, in press).

What is clear is that such a redefinition will be an essential prerequisite for any broad and sustainable change in policy and practice. We know, on the basis of both research and experience, that the poor health and early deaths of people with intellectual disabilities are not 'givens' and that they are (in part) preventable (Heslop et al., 2013; Krahn and Fox, in press; Mencap, 2012a). But there is a world of difference between recognising something as preventable and considering it intolerable to fail to prevent it. In short, we need to change the discourse about addressing the health inequalities experienced by people with intellectual disabilities from one based on improving the standards of public (and private) healthcare services to one based on the violation of the right of people with intellectual disabilities to health. We have no ready answers about how to bridge this gap, but potential avenues would include (but would not be confined to) the following two areas.

(1) **Generating more and better knowledge.** High-quality, up-to-date information on the scope and scale of issues relating to matters of social justice (and the extent of progress in addressing these issues) can help generate and maintain international, national and local political momentum. This is the core business of public health surveillance. Unfortunately (and as we have seen in this book), there is a paucity of good, credible, real-time information on the health inequalities faced by people with intellectual disabilities (or disabilities more generally). Whilst this is, in part, due to some important technical difficulties in collecting good surveillance data on people with intellectual disabilities (Centers for Disease Control and Prevention (CDC), 2011; Centers for Disease Control and Prevention (CDC) and National Center on Birth Defects and Developmental Disabilities (NCBDDD) Health Surveillance Work Group, 2009), it also reflects the low priority given to disabled people in public health (Emerson et al., 2011f) and (until recently) to health within intellectual disability research and practice. But this issue is about more than large-scale surveillance data. It also involves collecting and sharing information about people's experiences about what makes them ill and what happens to them when they become ill (Mencap, 2007, 2012a). Such information can have a powerful impact on public attitudes and political processes.

(2) **Creating alliances.** Three types of alliance may be particularly important. First, building alliances between the world of intellectual disability research/ practice and civil society organisations for (and sometimes run by) people with intellectual disabilities. Whilst the last decade has seen some significant small-scale developments in this area, there are few (if any) examples of sustainable large-scale alliances between intellectual disability research/

practice organisations and intellectual disability organisations. Second, building alliances between the world of intellectual disability research/practice and public health (Emerson et al., 2011f). Public health is paying increasing attention to the plight of marginalised or vulnerable social groups (World Health Organization, 2011a). A key task here is to help public health agencies understand that people with intellectual disabilities constitute an important marginalised or vulnerable segment of society that are at high risk of exposure to living conditions and experiences that are detrimental to their health. Third, building alliances between intellectual disability research/practice and general disability research/practice and policy organisations. The world of intellectual disability research is very insular. We rarely heed much attention to research looking at similar issues in the general population or amongst other groups of disabled people. Whilst the nature of impairment has an important impact on social responses to 'disability', there are likely to be times at which there would be significant value in working in alliance with others concerned with the well-being of disabled people more generally (World Health Organization and the World Bank, 2011).

A final word

Although we have included evidence from low- and middle-income countries where we can, this book has followed the vast bulk of the published research evidence and has largely focused on the public health of people with intellectual disabilities in high-income (and mainly English-speaking) countries (Emerson et al., 2007). We urgently need to develop a more balanced global perspective on the public health of people with intellectual disabilities for a number of reasons. Most obviously, the vast majority of people with intellectual disabilities with the greatest risk factors for poor health are likely to be living in low- and middle-income countries (Maulik et al., 2011; WHO, 2011b).

Furthermore, the profile of public health issues for people with intellectual disabilities in high-income countries is likely in many respects to be quite peculiar to these countries and not readily generalisable to low- and middle-income countries. Understanding more about the public health issues faced by people with intellectual disabilities in low- and middle-income countries will help us arrive at a much better understanding of how the social determinants of the health of people with intellectual disabilities play out in different social, political, economic, cultural and service contexts. It may also help us come up with a broader range of public health interventions towards the lower layers of the health impact pyramid (Figure 5.1) rather than focusing on health service responses to public health issues.

For example, while identifying people with intellectual disabilities in high-income countries relies on highly complex processes and classification criteria to be conducted by highly trained professionals (AAIDD, 2010), several less 'precise' but also less burdensome ways to screen for potential intellectual disability have been developed and used in low- and middle-income countries (see Roberts et al., 2012, for a systematic review). For public health surveillance purposes, such screening measures, conducted separately from complex assessments determining a person's eligibility for service support, may be a more productive way forward.

The dislocation of the 'hidden majority' of adults with intellectual disabilities from the minority of 'visible' adults with more severe intellectual disabilities known to specialist intellectual disability services may also only be a pressing issue in countries with particular service systems in place. Countries with service systems that do not provide such intensive service systems for a small proportion of adults with intellectual disabilities (with the consequent policing of eligibility boundaries) may have developed a range of different options for supporting adults with intellectual disabilities without specialist intellectual disability services which may be particularly valuable in public health terms. Ironically, although there are many obvious benefits of specialist intellectual disability services for those who receive/use them, in public health terms this book has demonstrated that even these specialist services are not particularly adept at promoting the health of those people with intellectual disabilities within them. Understanding the life course trajectories, socio-economic factors and public health interventions that promote positive health and reduce health inequalities for people with intellectual disabilities in the absence of comprehensive specialist intellectual disability services is vital if we are to take forward a serious public health agenda for all people with intellectual disabilities. This is no less an issue in high-income countries than in low- and middle-income countries, and can serve to connect us in our continuing quest for health equity for people with intellectual disabilities.

References

AAIDD. (2010). *Intellectual Disability: Definition, Classification, and Systems of Supports* (11th edn). Washington DC: AAIDD.

Abdullah, N., Drummond, P., Gray, N. et al. (2009). Short stature: Increased in children with severe learning disability. *Child: Care, Health and Development*, 35, 266–70.

Abu-Saad, K. and Fraser, D. (2010). Maternal nutrition and birth outcomes. *Epidemiologic Reviews*, 32, 5–25.

Ackers, R., Besag, F. M. C., Hughes, E. et al. (2011). Mortality rates and causes of death in children with epilepsy prescribed antiepileptic drugs. A retrospective cohort study using the UK General Practice Research Database. *Drug Safety*, 34(5), 403–13.

Adler, N. E. and Stewart, J. (2010). Health disparities across the lifespan: Meaning, methods, and mechanisms. *Annals of the New York Academy of Sciences*, 1186, 5–23.

Alborz, A., McNally, R. and Glendinning, C. (2005). Access to healthcare for people with learning disabilities in the UK: Mapping the issues and reviewing the evidence. *Journal of Health Services Research and Policy*, 10, 173–82.

Alborz, A., McNally, R. and Swallow, A. (2003). *From the Cradle to the Grave: A Literature Review of Access to Healthcare for People with Learning Disabilities across the Lifespan*. London: National Co-ordinating Centre for NHS Service Delivery and Organisation.

Alkire, S., Bastagli, F., Burchardt, T. et al. (2009). *Developing the Equality Measurement Framework: Selecting the Indicators*. Research Report 31. London.

Allerton, L. and Emerson, E. (Online early). Individuals with impairments face significant barriers to accessing health services in the United Kingdom. Public Health. DOI: http://dx.doi.org/10.1016/j.puhe.2012.08.003.

Almedom, A. M. (2005). Social capital and mental health: An interdisciplinary review of primary evidence. *Social Science and Medicine*, 61, 943–64.

Amark, K. and Sunnegardh, J. (1999). The effect of changing attitudes to Down's syndrome in the management of complete atrioventicular septal defects. *Archives of Disease in Childhood*, 81(2), 4.

Amiet, C., Gourfinkel-An, I., Bouzamondo, A. et al. (2008). Epilepsy in autism is associated with intellectual disability and gender: Evidence from a meta-analysis. *Biological Psychiatry*, 64, 577–82.

Anda, R. F., Felitti, V. J., Bremner, J. D. et al. (2006). The enduring effects of abuse and related adverse experiences in childhood: A convergence of evidence from neurobiology and epidemiology. *European Archives of Psychiatry and Clinical Neuroscience*, 256, 174–86.

Anders, P. L. (2010). Oral health of patients with intellectual disabilities: A systematic review. *Special Care in Dentistry*, 30(3), 8.

Andreias, L., Borawski, E., Schluchter, M. et al. (2010). Neighborhood influences on the academic achievement of extremely low birth weight children. *Journal of Pediatric Psychology*, 35, 275–83.

Annaz, D., Hill, C. M., Ashworth, A., Holley, S. and Karmiloff-Smith, A. (2011). Characterisation of sleep problems in children with Williams syndrome. *Research in Developmental Disabilities*, 32, 164–9.

Arron, K., Oliver, C., Moss, J., Berg, K. and Burbidge, C. (2011). The prevalence and phenomenology of self-injurious and aggressive behaviour in genetic syndromes. *Journal of Intellectual Disability Research*, 55, 109–20.

Arseneault, L., Bowes, L. and Shakoor, S. (2010). Bullying victimization in youths and mental health problems: 'Much ado about nothing'? *Psychological Medicine*, 40, 717–29.

Arshad, S., Winterhalder, R., Underwood, L. et al. (2011). Epilepsy and intellectual disability: Does epilepsy increase the likelihood of co-morbid psychopathology? *Research in Developmental Disabilities*, 32, 353–7.

Audit Commission. (2007). *Out of Authority Placements for Special Educational Needs*. London: Audit Commission.

Australian Institute of Health and Welfare. (2012). *Australia's Health 2012*. Canberra: Australian Institute of Health and Welfare.

Azmi, S., Hatton, C., Emerson, E. and Caine, A. (1997). Listening to adolescents and adults with intellectual disabilities from South Asian communities. *Journal of Applied Research in Intellectual Disabilities*, 10, 250–63.

Baird, P. A. and Sadovnick, A. D. (1988). Life expectancy in Down syndrome adults. *Lancet*, 332, 1354–6.

Ball, S. L., Panter, S. G., Redley, M. et al. (2012). The extent and nature of need for mealtime support among adults with intellectual disabilities. *Journal of Intellectual Disability Research*, 56, 382–401.

Balogh, R., Brownell, M., Ouellette-Kuntz, H. and Colantonio, A. (2010). Hospitalisation rates for ambulatory care-sensitive conditions for persons with and without an intellectual disability – a population perspective. *Journal of Intellectual Disability Research*, 54, 820–32.

Balogh, R., Hunter, D. and Ouellette-Kuntz, H. (2005). Hospital utilization among persons with an intellectual disability, Ontario, Canada, 1995–2001. *Journal of Applied Research in Intellectual Disabilities*, 18, 181–90.

Balogh, R. S., Ouellette-Kuntz, H., Brownell, M. and Colantonio, A. (2013). Factors associated with hospitalisations for ambulatory care-sensitive conditions among persons with an intellectual disability – a publicly insured population perspective. *Journal of Intellectual Disabilities Research*, 57, 226–39.

Bambra, C., Gibson, M., Sowden, A. et al. (2010). Tackling the wider social determinants of health and health inequalities: Evidence from systematic reviews. *Journal of Epidemiology and Community Health*, 64, 284–91.

Barger, E., Wacker, J., Macy, R., Parish, S. (2009). Sexual assault prevention for women with intellectual disabilities: a critical review of the evidence. *Intellectual and Developmental Disabilities*, 47(4), 14.

Barnes, C. (2012). Understanding the social model of disability: Past, present and future. In N. Watson, A. Roulstone and C. Thomas (eds.), *Routledge Handbook of Disability Studies*. Abingdon: Routledge, pp. 12–29.

Barr, O., Gilgunn, J., Kane, T. and Moore, G. (1999). Health screening for people with learning disabilities by a community learning disability nursing service in Northern Ireland. *Journal of Advanced Nursing*, 29(6), 1482–91.

Barros, F. C., Matijasevich, A., Requejo, J. H. et al. (2010). Recent trends in maternal, newborn, and child health in Brazil: Progress toward Millennium Development Goals 4 and 5. *American Journal of Public Health*, 100, 1877–89.

Bartley, M. (2004). *Health Inequality*. Cambridge: Polity Press.

Bartlo, P. and Klein, P. J. (2011). Physical activity benefits and needs in adults with intellectual disabilities: Systematic review of the literature. *American Journal of Intellectual and Developmental Disabilities*, 116, 220–32.

Bastiaanse, L. P., Hilgenkamp, T. I. M., Echteld, M. A. and Evenhuis, H. M. (2012). Prevalence and associated factors of sarcopenia in older adults with intellectual disabilities. *Research in Developmental Disabilities*, 33, 2004–12.

Batshaw, M. L., Pellegrino, L. and Roizen, N. J. (eds.). (2007). *Children with Disabilities* (6th edition). Baltimore, MD: P. H. Brookes.

Batty, G. D., Deary, I. J. and Gottfredson, L. S. (2007). Premorbid (early life) IQ and later mortality risk: Systematic review. *Annals of Epidemiology*, 17(4), 278–88.

Batty, G. D., Der, G., Macintyre, S. and Deary, I. J. (2006). Does IQ explain socio-economic inequalities in health? Evidence from a population-based cohort study in the west of Scotland. *British Medical Journal*, 332, 580–4.

Batty, G. D., Gale, C. R., Tynelius, P., Deary, I. J. and Rasmussen, F. (2009). IQ in early adulthood, socio-economic position, and unintentional injury mortality by middle age: A cohort study of more than 1 million Swedish men. *American Journal of Epidemiology*, 169(5), 606–15.

Baxter, H., Lowe, K., Houston, H. et al. (2006). Previously unidentified morbidity in patients with intellectual disability. *British Journal of General Practice*, 56(523), 93–8.

Beange, H., McElduff, A. and Baker, W. (1995). Medical disorders of adults with mental retardation: A population study. *American Journal on Mental Retardation*, 99, 595–604.

Beecham, J., Chadwick, O., Fidan, D. and Bernard, S. (2002). Children with severe learning disabilities: Needs, services and costs. *Children and Society*, 16, 168–81.

Bell, A. and Bhate, M. (1992). Prevalence of overweight and obesity in Down's syndrome and other mentally handicapped adults living in the community. *Journal of Intellectual Disability Research*, 36, 359–64.

Belva, B. C., Matson, J. L., Sipes, M. and Bamburg, J. W. (2012). An examination of specific communication deficits in adults with profound intellectual disabilities. *Research in Developmental Disabilities*, 33, 525–9.

Bengtsson, S., Hansen, H. and Røgeskov, M. (2011). *Børn med en funktionsnedsættelse og deres familier* [Children with disabilities and their families]. Report 11:09. Copenhagen: Danish National Centre for Social Research.

Bernal, J. (2008). Telling the truth or not: Disclosure and information for people with intellectual disabilities who have cancer. *International Journal on Disability and Human Development*, 7, 365–70.

Bershadsky, J., Taub, S., Engler, S. (2012). Place of residence and preventive health care for intellectual and developmental disabilities services recipients in 20 states. *Public Health Reports*, 127(5), 11.

Berry, J. G., Bloom, S., Foley, S. and Palfrey, J. S. (2010). Health inequity in children and youth with chronic health conditions. *Pediatrics*, 126, S111–19. DOI: 10.1542/peds.2010-1466D.

Bhaumik, S., Watson, J. M., Thorp, C. F., Tyrer, F. and McGrother, C. W. (2008). Body mass index in adults with intellectual disability: Distribution, associations and service implications: A population-based prevalence study. *Journal of Intellectual Disability Research*, 52, 287–98.

Bickenbach, J. E. (2012). The International Classification of Functioning, Disability and Health and its relationship to disability studies. In N. Watson, A. Roulstone and C. Thomas (eds.), *Routledge Handbook of Disability Studies*. London: Routledge, (pp. 51–66).

Bigby, C. (2008). Known well by no one: Trends in the informal social networks of middle-aged and older people with intrellectual disability five years after moving to the community. *Journal of Intellectual and Developmental Disability*, 33, 148–57.

Bittles, A. H., Petterson, B. A., Sullivan, S. G., Hussain, R., Glasson, E. J. and Montgomery, P. (2002). The influence of intellectual disability on life expectancy. *Journal of Geron-tology*, 57, 470–2.

Blacher, J. and Begum, G. F. (2011). Sibling relationship quality and adjustment: Considerations of family, genetics, cultural expectations and disability types. In R. Hodapp (ed.), *International Review of Research in Developmental Disability, Volume 41*. Chennai, India: Elsevier, pp. 163–97.

Blacher, J., Begum, G., Marcoulides, G. and Baker, B. L. (in press). Longitudinal perspectives of child-positive impact on families: Relationship to disability and culture. *American Journal of Intellectual and Developmental Disabilities*.

Black, R. E., Allen, L. H., Bhutta, Z. A. et al. (2008). Maternal and child undernutrition: Global and regional exposures and health consequences. *Lancet*, 371, 243–60.

Black, R. E., Morris, S. S. and Bryce, J. (2003). Where and why are 10 million children dying every year? *Lancet*, 361, 2226–34.

Böhmer, C. J., Niezen-de Boer, M. C., Klinkenberg-Knol, E. C. et al. (1999). The prevalence of gastroesophageal reflux disease in institutionalized intellectually disabled individuals. *American Journal of Gastroenterology*, 94, 804–10.

Böhmer, C. J., Taminiau, J. A., Klinkenberg-Knol, E. C. and Meuwissen, S. G. (2001). The prevalence of constipation in institutionalized people with intellectual disability. *Journal of Intellectual Disability Research*, 45, 212–18.

Bolte, G., Tamburlini, G. and Kohlhuber, M. (2010). Environmental inequalities among children in Europe: Evaluation of scientific evidence and policy implications. *European Journal of Public Health*, 20, 14–20.

Bonell, S. (2010). Neoplasms. In J. O'Hara, J. E. McCarthy and N. Bouras (eds.), *Intellectual Disability and Ill Health: A Review of the Evidence*. Cambridge University Press, pp. 127–36.

Bouras, N. and Holt, G. (eds.). (2007). *Psychiatric and Behavioural Disorders in Intellectual and Developmental Disabilities*. Cambridge University Press.

Boyle, A., Melville, C. A., Morrison, J. et al. (2010). A cohort study of the prevalence of sleep problems in adults with intellectual disabilities. *Journal of Sleep Research*, 19, 42–53.

Branford, D., Bhaumik, S. and Duncan, F. (1998). Epilepsy in adults with learning disabilities. *Seizure*, 7, 473–7.

Braubach, M. and Fairburn, J. (2010). Social inequities in environmental risks associated with housing and residential location: A review of evidence. *European Journal of Public Health*, 20, 36–42.

Breau, L. M., Camfield, C. S., McGrath, P. J. and Finley, G. A. (2007). Pain's impact on adaptive functioning. *Journal of Intellectual Disability Research*, 51, 125–34.

Breau, L. M., MacLaren, J., McGrath, P. J., Camfield, C. S. and Finlay, W. M. (2003). Caregivers' beliefs regarding pain in children with cognitive impairment: Relation between pain sensation and reaction increases with severity of impairment. *Clinical Journal of Pain*, 19, 335–44.

Brickman, P. and Campbell, D. T. (1971). Hedonic relativism and planning the good society. In M. H. Apley (ed.), *Adaptation-Level Theory: A Symposium*. New York: Academic Press, pp. 287–302.

Brookes, M. E. and Alberman, E. (1996). Early mortality and morbidity in children with Down's syndrome diagnosed in two regional health authorities in 1988. *Journal of Medical Screening*, 3, 7–11.

Brown, L. F. (1994). Research in dental health education and health promotion: A review of the literature. *Health Education Quarterly*, 21(1), 20.

Brown, S., Kim, M., Mitchell, C. and Inskip, H. (2010). Twenty-five-year mortality of a community cohort with schizophrenia. *British Journal of Psychiatry*, 196(2), 116–21. DOI: 10.1192/bjp.bp.109.067512.

Bruce, N., Pope, D. and Stanistreet, D. (2008). Standardisation. In N. Bruce, D. Pope and D. Stanistreet (eds.), *Quantitative Methods for Health Research: A Practical Interactive Guide to Epidemiology and Statistics*. Chichester: John Wiley and Sons, pp. 111–28.

Brukiene, V. and Aleksejuniene, J. (2009). An overview of oral health promotion in adolescence. *International Journal of Paediatric Dentistry*, 19(3), 9.

Buntinx, W. H. E. and Schalock, R. L. (2010). Models of disability, quality of life, and individualized supports: implications for professional practice in intellectual disability. *Journal of Policy and Practice in Intellectual Disabilities*, 7(4), 283–294.

Burchardt, T. (2004). Capabilities and disability: The capabilities framework and the social model of disability. *Disability and Society*, 19(7), 735–51.

Burchardt, T. (2008). Monitoring inequality: Putting the capability approach to work. In G. Craig, T. Burchardt and D. Gordon (eds.), *Social Justice and Public Policy*. Bristol: Policy Press, pp. 205–29.

Burchardt, T., & Vizard, P. (2011). 'Operationalizing' the capability approach as a basis for equality and human rights monitoring in twenty-first-century Britain. *Journal of Human Development and Capabilities*, 12(1), 91–119.

Bzostek, S. H. and Beck, A. N. (2011). Familial instability and young children's physical health. *Social Science and Medicine*, 73, 282–92.

Calders, P. E., Elmahgoub, S., de Mettelinge, T. R. et al. (2011). Effect of combined exercise training on physical and metabolic fitness in adults with intellectual disability: A controlled trial. *Clinical Rehabilitation*, 25(12), 12.

Calvin, C. M., Deary, I. J., Fenton, C. et al. (2011). Intelligence in youth and all-cause-mortality: Systematic review with meta-analysis. *International Journal of Epidemiology*, 40, 626–44.

Campbell, V. A. and Fedeyko, H. J. (2001). The healthy people 2010 process. In A. J. Tymchuk, C. Lakin and R. Luckasson (eds.), *The Forgotten Generation: The Status and Challenges of Adults with Mild Cognitive Limitations*. Baltimore, MD: Paul H Brookes, pp. 221–46.

Cardoza, B. and Kerr, M. (2010). Diseases of the nervous system I: Epilepsy, hydroceophalus and nervous system malformations. In J. O'Hara, J. E. McCarthy and N. Bouras (eds.), *Intellectual Disability and Ill Health: A Review of the Evidence*. Cambridge University Press, pp. 190–202.

Care Quality Commission. (2012). *Learning Disability Services Inspection Programme: National Overview*. London: Care Quality Commission.

Carlsen, W. R. and Galluzzi, K. E. (1994). Comprehensive geriatric assessment: Applications for community-residing elderly people with mental retardation/developmental disabilities. *Mental Retardation*, 32(5), 334.

Carmeli, E., Imamb, B., Bachar, A. and Merrick, J. (2012). Inflammation and oxidative stress as biomarkers of premature aging in persons with intellectual disability. *Research in Developmental Disabilities*, 33, 369–75.

Carpenter, G. L. and Stacks, A. M. (2009). Developmental effects of exposure to Intimate Partner Violence in early childhood: A review of the literature. *Children and Youth Services Review*, 31, 831–9.

Carter, M., McCaughey, E., Annaz, D. and Hill, C. M. (2009). Sleep problems in a Down syndrome population. *Archives of Disease in Childhood*, 94, 308–10.

Carter, M., Parmenter, T. and Watters, M. (2006). National, metropolitan and local newsprint coverage of developmental disibility. *Journal of Intellectual and Developmental Disability*, 21, 173–98.

Carvill, S. (2001). Review: Sensory impairments, intellectual disability and psychiatry. *Journal of Intellectual Disability Research*, 45, 467–83.

Cassidy, G., Martin, D. M., Martin, G. H. B. and Roy, A. (2002). Health checks for people with learning disabilities: Community learning disability teams working with general practitioners and primary healthcare teams. *Journal of Learning Disabilities (14690047)*, 6(2), 123–36.

Caton, S., Chadwick, D., Chapman, M. et al. (2012). Healthy lifestyles for adults with intellectual disability: Knowledge, barriers, and facilitators. *Journal of Intellectual and Developmental Disability*, 37, 248–59.

Center, J., Beange, H. and McElduff, A. (1998). People with mental retardation have an increased prevalence of osteoporosis: A population study. *American Journal on Mental Retardation*, 103, 19–28.

Centers for Disease Control and Prevention (CDC). (2011). *CDC Health Disparities and Inequalities Report – United States, 2011*. Atlanta: Centers for Disease Control and Prevention.

Centers for Disease Control and Prevention (CDC) and National Center on Birth Defects and Developmental Disabilities (NCBDDD) Health Surveillance Work Group. (2009). *U.S. Surveillance of Health of People with Intellectual Disabilities*. Atlanta: CDC/ NCBDDD.

Chadwick, D. and Jolliffe, J. (2009). A descriptive investigation of dysphagia in adults with intellectual disabilities. *Journal of Intellectual Disability Research*, 53, 29–43.

Chapman, D., Scott, K. and Stanton-Chapman, T. (2008). Public health approach to the study of mental retardation. *American Journal on Mental Retardation*, 113(2), 102–16.

Chapman, M., Iddon, P., Atkinson, K. et al. (2010). The misdiagnosis of epilepsy in people with intellectual disabilities: A systematic review. *Seizure*, 20, 101–6.

Chapman, S. L. C. and Wu, T. (2012). Substance abuse among individuals with intellectual disabilities. *Research in Developmental Disabilities*, 33, 1147–56.

Chauhan, U., Reeve, J., Kontopantelis, E. et al. (2012). *Impact of the English Directly Enhanced Service (DES) for Learning Disability*. Manchester: Health Sciences Research Group, University of Manchester.

Chen, C., Hsu, K., Shu, B. and Fetzer, S. (2012). The image of people with intellectual disability in Taiwan newspapers. *Journal of Intellectual and Developmental Disability*, 37, 35–41.

Chin, H. B., Sipe, T. A., Elder, R., Mercer, S. L., Chattopadhyay, S. K., Jacob, V., Task, C. P. S. (2012). The effectiveness of group-based comprehensive risk-reduction and abstinence education interventions to prevent or reduce the risk of adolescent pregnancy, human immunodeficiency virus, and sexually transmitted infections two systematic reviews for the guide to community preventive services. *American Journal of Preventive Medicine,* 42(3), 272–294.

Choi, E., Park, H., Ha, Y. and Hwang, W. J. (2012). Prevalence of overweight and obesity in children with intellectual disabilities in Korea. *Journal of Applied Research in Intellectual Disabilities,* 25, 476–83.

Claes, C., Van Hove, G., van Loon, J., Vandevelde, S., & Schalock, R. L. (2010). Quality of life measurement in the field of intellectual disabilities: eight principles for assessing quality of life-related personal outcomes. *Social Indicators Research,* 98(1), 61–72.

Clarke, D., Vemuri, M., Gunatilake, D. and Tewari, S. (2008). Helicobacter pylori infection in five inpatient units for people with intellectual disability and psychiatric disorder. *Journal of Applied Research in Intellectual Disabilities,* 21(1), 95–8.

Cockerell, O. C., Johnson, A. L., Sander, J. W. A. S. et al. (1994). Mortality from epilepsy: Results from a prospective population-based study. *Lancet,* 344(8927), 918.

Coleman, J. and Spurling, G. (2010). Easily missed? Constipation in people with learning disability. *BMJ,* 340(7745), 531.

Commission on Funding of Care and Support. (2011). *Fairer Care Funding: Analysis and Evidence Supporting the Recommendations of the Commission on Funding of Care and Support London.*

Conger, R. D. and Donnellan, M. B. (2007). An interactionist perspective on the socio-economic context of human development. *Annual Review of Psychology,* 58, 175–99.

Cooke, L. B. (1997). Cancer and learning disability. *Journal of Intellectual Disability Research,* 41, 312–16.

Cooper, S. A. (1997a). Deficient health and social services for elderly people with learning disabilities. *Journal of Intellectual Disability Research,* 41, 331–8.

Cooper, S. A. (1997b). High prevalence of dementia among people with learning disabilities not attributable to Down's syndrome. *Psychological Medicine,* 27, 609–16.

Cooper, S. A. (1997c). A population-based health survey of maladaptive behaviours associated with dementia in elderly people with learning disabilities. *Journal of Intellectual Disability Research,* 41, 481–7.

Cooper, S. A. (2004). Mental health. In E. Emerson, C. Hatton, T. Thompson and T. Parmenter (eds.), *International Handbook of Applied Research in Intellectual Disabilities.* Chichester: Wiley, pp. 407–22.

Cooper, S. A., McConnachie, A., Allan, L. M. et al. (2011). Neighbourhood deprivation, health inequalities and service access by adults with intellectual disabilities: A cross-sectional study. *Journal of Intellectual Disability Research,* 55, 313–23.

Cooper, S. A., Morrison, J., Melville, C. et al. (2006). Improving the health of people with intellectual disabilities: Outcomes of a health screening programme after 1 year. *Journal of Intellectual Disability Research,* 50, 667–77. DOI: 10.1111/j.1365-2788.2006.00824.x.

Cooper, S. A., Smiley, E., Allan, L. et al. (2009a). Adults with intellectual disabilities: Prevalence, incidence and remission of self-injurious behaviour and related factors. *Journal of Intellectual Disability Research,* 53, 200–16.

Cooper, S. A., Smiley, E., Finlayson, J. et al. (2007a). The prevalence, incidence and factors predictive of mental ill-health in adults with profound intellectual disabilities. *Journal of Applied Research in Intellectual Disabilities,* 20, 493–501.

Cooper, S. A., Smiley, E., Jackson, A. et al. (2009b). Adults with intellectual disabilities: Prevalence, incidence and remission of aggressive behaviour and related factors. *Journal of Intellectual Disability Research*, 53, 217–32.

Cooper, S. A., Smiley, E., Morrison, J., Williamson, A. and Allan, L. (2007b). Mental ill-health in adults with intellectual disabilities: Prevalence and associated factors. *British Journal of Psychiatry*, 190, 27–35.

Cooper, S. A. J. (2003). The Diagnostic Criteria for Psychiatric Disorders for Use with Adults with Learning Disabilities (DC-LD) papers. *Journal of Intellectual Disabilities Research*, 47(Suppl. 1), 1–2.

Copeland, A. and Glover, G. (2012). *Autism Self-Assessment Framework 2011: Initial Findings*. Durham: Improving Health and Lives: Learning Disabilities Observatory.

Copeland, A., McLean, J. and Glover, G. (2012). *Local Authority Self-assessment of Services for People with Autism in 2010/2011 – Ratings Atlas*. Durham: Improving Health and Lives: Learning Disabilities Public Health Observatory.

Coppus, A. M., Evenhuis, H. M., Verberne, G. J. et al. (2006). Dementia and mortality in persons with Down syndrome. *Journal of Intellectual Disabilities Research*, 50, 768–77.

Coppus, A. M., Evenhuis, H. M., Verberne, G. J. et al. (2008). Survival in elderly persons with Down syndrome. *Journal of the American Geriatrics Society*, 56, 2311–16.

Coppus, A. M. W., Evenhuis, H. M., Verberne, G. J. et al. (2010). Early age at menopause is associated with increased risk of dementia and mortality in women with Down syndrome. *Journal of Alzheimer's Disease*, 19, 545–50.

Croen, L. A., Grether, J. K. and Selvin, S. (2001). The epidemiology of mental retardation of unknown cause. *Pediatrics*, 107 e86, 1–5.

Crombie, H., Killoran, A. and Naidoo, B. (2010). What environmental changes can increase physical activity? In A. Killoran and M. P. Kelly (eds.), *Evidence-based Public Health: Effectiveness and Efficiency*. Oxford University Press, pp. 382–97.

Cummins, R. (2002). Proxy responding for subjective well-being: A review. In L. M. Glidden (ed.), *International Review of Research in Mental Retardation, Vol. 25*. San Diego, CA: Academic Press, pp. 183–207.

Cummins, R. (2003). Normative life satisfaction: Measurement issues and a homeostatic model. *Social Indicators Research*, 64(2), 225–56.

Cummins, S. (2010). Improving population health through area-based social interventions. In A. Killoran and M. P. Kelly (eds.), *Evidence-based Public Health: Effectiveness and Efficiency*. Oxford University Press, pp. 287–97.

Dagnan, D. (2007). Commentary: the prevalence, incidence and factors predictive of mental ill-health in adults with profound intellectual disabilities. *Journal of Applied Research in Intellectual Disabilities*, 20, 502–4.

Dagnan, D. and Lindsay, W. R. (2012). People with intellectual disabilities and mental ill health. In E. Emerson, C. Hatton, K. Dickson, R. Gone, A. Caine and J. Bromley (eds.), *Clinical Psychology and People with Intellectual Disabilities*. Chichester: Wiley, pp. 313–38.

Dahlgren, G. and Whitehead, M. (1991/2007). Policies and strategies to promote social equity in health. Background document to WHO – Strategy paper for Europe (www.framtidsstudier.se/wp-content/uploads/2011/01/20080109110739filmZ8UVQv2wQFShMRF6cuT.pdf). Stockholm: Institutet för Framtidsstudier.

Daly, A. (2006). *Social Inclusion and Exclusion among Australia's Children: A Review of the Literature*. Canberra: National Centre for Social and Economic Modelling, University of Canberra.

Das, M., Spowart, K., Crossley, S. and Dutton, G. N. (2010). Evidence that children with special needs all require visual assessment. *Archive of Diseases of Childhood*, 95, 888–92.

Davey Smith, G. (ed.). (2002). *Health Inequalities: Life Course Approaches*. Bristol: Policy Press.

Davey Smith, G., Dorling, D. and Shaw, M. (eds.). (2001). *Poverty, Inequality and Health in Britain 1800–2000: A Reader*. Bristol: Policy Press.

Davies, G. (2012). *Oral Health among Adults with Learning Disabilities in England 2010/11*. Paper presented at Better Dental Services for People with Learning Disabilities, Birmingham.

Davies, N. and Duff, M. (2001). Breast cancer screening for older women with intellectual disability living in community group homes. *Journal of Intellectual Disability Research*, 45, 253–7.

Davis, R. W. (2010). Digestive system diseases. In J. O'Hara, J. E. McCarthy and N. Bouras (eds.), *Intellectual Disability and Ill Health: A Review of the Evidence*. Cambridge University Press, pp. 88–97.

Davydov, D., Stewart, R., Ritchie, K. and Chaudieu, I. (2010). Resilience and mental health. *Clinical Psychology Review*, 30, 479–95.

de Kuijper, G., Hoekstra, P., Visser, F. et al. (2010). Use of antipsychotic drugs in individuals with intellectual disability (ID) in the Netherlands: Prevalence and reasons for prescription. *Journal of Intellectual Disability Research*, 54, 659–67.

Denis, C., Lavie, E., Fatseas, M., Auriacombe, M. (2006). Psychotherapeutic interventions for cannabis abuse and/or dependence in outpatient settings: Cochrane Database of Systematic Reviews.

de Winter, C. F., Bastiaanse, L. P., Hilgenkamp, T. I. M., Evenhuis, H. M. and Echteld, M. A. (2012a). Cardiovascular risk factors (diabetes, hypertension, hypercholesterolemia and metabolic syndrome) in older people with intellectual disability: Results of the HA-ID study. *Research in Developmental Disabilities*, 33, 1722–31.

de Winter, C. F., Bastiaanse, L. P., Hilgenkamp, T. I. M., Evenhuis, H. M. and Echteld, M. A. (2012b). Overweight and obesity in older people with intellectual disability. *Research in Developmental Disabilities*, 33, 398–405.

Department for Education. (2012). *Support and Aspiration: A New Approach to Special Educational Needs and Disability – Progress and Next Steps*. London: Department for Education.

Department for Work and Pensions. (2013). *Fulfilling Potential: Building a Deeper Understanding of Disability in the UK Today*. London: Department for Work and Pensions.

Department of Developmental Services. (2011). *Mortality Annual Report FY 2010*. Department of Developmental Services.

Department of Developmental Services. (2012). *Mortality Annual Report FY 2011*. Department of Developmental Services.

Department of Health. (2007). *Services for People with Learning Disabilities and Challenging Behaviour or Mental Health Needs (Revised Edition)*. London: Department of Health.

Department of Health (2009). *Learning Disabilities Positive Practice Guide*. London: Department of Health.

Department of Health. (2010a). *Healthy Lives, Healthy People: Our Strategy for Public Health in England*. London: Department of Health.

Department of Health. (2010b). *Prioritising Need in the Context of Putting People First. A Whole System Approach to Eligibility for Social Care: Guidance on Eligibility Criteria for Adult Social Care, England 2010*. London: Department of Health.

Department of Health. (2011). *Victorian Population Health Survey of People with an Intellectual Disability 2009*. Melbourne: State Government of Victoria.

Department of Health. (2012a). *NHS Outcomes Framework: A Technical Annex about Setting Levels of Ambition* (Chapter 3 part 2, section 1.7). Gateway reference 17770. London: Department of Health. Available online at www.dh.gov.uk/health/2012/07/nhsof-levels-ambition.

Department of Health. (2012b). *Transforming Care: A National Response to Winterbourne View Hospital. Final Report*. London: Department of Health.

Department of Health. (2012c). *Winterbourne View Review. Concordat: Programme of Action*. London: Department of Health.

DeSalvo, K. B., Bloser, N., Reynolds, K., He, J. and Muntner, P. (2006). Mortality prediction with a single general self-rated health question: A meta-analysis. *Journal of General Internal Medicine*, 21, 267–75.

DeWalt, D. A. and Hink, A. (2009). Health literacy and child health outcomes: A systematic review of the literature. *Pediatrics*, 124(Suppl. 3), S265–74.

Dias, S., Ware, R. S., Kinner, S. A. and Lennox, N. (in press). Physical health outcomes in prisoners with intellectual disability: A cross-sectional study. *Journal of Intellectual Disabilities Research*.

Dickson, K., Emerson, E. and Hatton, C. (2005). Self-reported anti-social behaviour: Prevalence and risk factors amongst adolescents with and without intellectual disability. *Journal of Intellectual Disability Research*, 49, 820–6.

Diener, E. and Biswas-Diener, R. (2008). *Happiness: Unlocking the Mysteries of Psychological Wealth*. Oxford: Wiley-Blackwell.

Dinsmore, A. P. (2011). A small-scale investigation of hospital experiences among people with a learning disability on Merseyside: Speaking with patients and their carers. *British Journal of Learning Disabilities*, 40, 201–12.

Disability Rights Commission. (2006). *Equal Treatment – Closing the Gap*. London: Disability Rights Commission.

Djuretic, T., Laing-Morton, T., Guy, M. and Gill, M. (1999). Concerted effort is needed to ensure these women use preventive services. *British Medical Journal*, 318, 536.

Dobbins M., De Corby K., Robeson P., Husson H., Tirilis D. (2009). School-based physical activity programs for promoting physical activity and fitness in children and adolescents aged 6–18. *Cochrane Database of Systematic Reviews*, Issue 1. Art. No.: CD007651. DOI: 10.1002/14651858.CD007651.

Doughty, A. H. and Kane, L. M. (2010). Teaching abuse-protection skills to people with intellectual disabilities: A review of the literature. *Research in Developmental Disabilities*, 31, 331–7.

Douglas, N. A. (2010). Infectious diseases. In J. O'Hara, J. E. McCarthy and N. Bouras (eds.), *Intellectual Disability and Ill Health: A Review of the Evidence*. Cambridge University Press, pp. 47–60.

Drum, C. E., Krahn, G.-L. and Bersani H. (eds.). (2009). *Disability and Public Health*. Washington, DC: American Public Health Association.

Duff, M., Hoghton, M., Scheepers, M., Cooper, M. and Baddeley, P. (2001). Helicobacter pylori: Has the killer escaped from the institution? A possible cause of increased stomach cancer in a population with intellectual disability. *Journal of Intellectual Disability Research*, 45, 219–25.

Duke, T., Keshishiyan, E., Kuttumuratova, A. et al. (2006). Quality of hospital care for children in Kazakhstan, Republic of Moldova, and Russia: Systematic observational assessment. *Lancet*, 376(9514), 919–25.

Dukes, E.; McGuire, B.E. (2009). Enhancing capacity to make sexuality-related decisions in people with an intellectual disability. *Journal of Intellectual Disability Research*, 53(8), 8.

Duncan, G. J. and Brooks-Gunn, J. (2000). Family poverty, welfare reform, and child development. *Child Development*, 71, 188–96.

Duncan, G. J., Brooks-Gunn, J. and Klebanov, P. K. (1994). Economic deprivation and early childhood development. *Child Development*, 65, 296–318.

Durkin, M. (2002). The epidemiology of developmental disabilities in low-income countries. *Mental Retardation and Developmental Disabilities Research Reviews*, 8(3), 206–11.

Dykens, E. M., Hodapp, R. M. and Finucane, B. M. (2000). *Genetics and Mental Retardation Syndromes: A New Look at Behavior and Interventions*. Baltimore, MD: Paul H. Brookes Publishing.

Eayres, D. (2008). *Commonly Used Public Health Statistics and Their Confidence Intervals*. York: Association of Public Health Observatories.

Edgerton, R. B. (2001). The hidden majority of individuals with mental retardation or developmental disabilities. In A. J. Tymchuk, K. C. Lakin and R. Luckasson (eds.), *The Forgotten Generation: The Status and Challenges of Adults with Mild Cognitive Limitations*. Baltimore, MD: Brookes.

Einfeld, S., Ellis, L. and Emerson, E. (2011). Comorbidity of intellectual disability and mental disorder: A systematic review. *Journal of Intellectual and Developmental Disability*, 36, 137–43.

Einfeld, S. and Emerson, E. (2008). Intellectual disability. In M. Rutter, D. Bishop, D. Pine, S. Scott, J. Stevenson, E. Taylor and A. Thapar (eds.), *Rutter's Child and Adolescent Psychiatry* (5th edn). Oxford: Blackwell.

Einfeld, S. L. and Tonge, B. J. (1999). Observations on the use of the ICD-10 Guide for Mental Retardation. *Journal of Intellectual Disability Research*, 43, 408–13.

Elliott, J., Hatton, C. and Emerson, E. (2003). The health of people with learning disabilities in the UK: Evidence and implications for the NHS. *Journal of Integrated Care*, 11, 9–17.

Elmahgoub, S. M. L., Lambers, S., Stegen, S. et al. (2009). The influence of combined exercise training on indices of obesity, physical fitness and lipid profile in overweight and obese adolescents with mental retardation. *European Journal of Pediatrics*, 168, 1327–33.

Elsabbagh, M., Divan, G., Koh, Y. et al. (2012). Global prevalence of autism and other pervasive developmental disorders. *Autism Research*, 5, 160–79.

Emerson, E. (2003). Prevalence of psychiatric disorders in children and adolescents with and without intellectual disability. *Journal of Intellectual Disability Research*, 47, 51–8.

Emerson, E. (2005a). Underweight, obesity and physical activity in adults with intellectual disability in supported accommodation in Northern England. *Journal of Intellectual Disability Research*, 49, 134–43.

Emerson, E. (2005b). Use of the strengths and difficulties questionnaire to assess the mental health needs of children and adolescents with intellectual disabilities. *Journal of Intellectual and Developmental Disability*, 30, 14–23.

Emerson, E. (2007). Poverty and people with intellectual disability. *Mental Retardation and Developmental Disabilities Research Reviews*, 13, 107–13.

Emerson, E. (2009). Overweight and obesity in 3 and 5 year-old children with and without developmental delay. *Public Health*, 123, 130–3.

Emerson, E. (2010). Self-reported exposure to disablism is associated with poorer self-reported health and well-being among adults with intellectual disabilities in England: Cross-sectional survey. *Public Health*, 124(12), 682–9.

Emerson, E. (2011). Health status and health risks of the 'hidden majority' of adults with intellectual disability. *Intellectual and Developmental Disabilities*, 49, 155–65.

Emerson, E. (2012a). Deprivation, ethnicity and the prevalence of intellectual and developmental disabilities. *Journal of Epidemiology and Community Health*, 66(3), 218–24.

Emerson, E. (2012b). *A Review of the Results of the 2011/12 Focused CQC Inspection of Services for People with Learning Disabilities*. Durham: Improving Health and Lives: Learning Disabilities Observatory.

Emerson, E. (2012c). Understanding disabled childhoods: What can we learn from population-based studies? *Children and Society*, 26, 214–22.

Emerson, E. (Online early). Commentary: Childhood exposure to environmental adversity and the well-being of people with intellectual disabilities. *Journal of Intellectual Disabilities Research*. DOI: 10.1111/j.1365-2788.2012.01577.x.

Emerson, E., Baines, S., Allerton, L. and Welch, V. (2011a). *Health Inequalities and People with Learning Disabilities in the UK: 2011*. Durham: Improving Health and Lives: Learning Disabilities Observatory.

Emerson, E., Baines, S., Allerton, L. and Welch, V. (2012a). *Health Inequalities and People with Learning Disabilities in the UK: 2012*. Durham: Improving Health and Lives: Learning Disabilities Observatory.

Emerson, E. and Einfeld, S. (2010). Emotional and behavioural difficulties in young children with and without developmental delay: A bi-national perspective. *Journal of Child Psychology and Psychiatry*, 51, 583–93.

Emerson, E. and Einfeld, S. (2011). *Challenging Behaviour* (3rd edn). Cambridge University Press.

Emerson, E., Einfeld, S. and Stancliffe, R. (2010). The mental health of young Australian children with intellectual disabilities or borderline intellectual functioning. *Social Psychiatry and Psychiatric Epidemiology*, 45, 579–87.

Emerson, E., Einfeld, S. and Stancliffe, R. J. (2011b). Predictors of the persistence of conduct difficulties in children with cognitive delay. *Journal of Child Psychology and Psychiatry and Allied Disciplines*, 52, 1184–94.

Emerson, E., Felce, D. and Stancliffe, R. (in press). Issues concerning self-report data and population-based data sets involving people with intellectual disabilities. Intellectual and Developmental Disabilities.

Emerson, E., Fujiura, G. T. and Hatton, C. (2007). International perspectives. In S. L. Odom, R. H. Horner, M. Snell and J. Blacher (eds.), *Handbook on Developmental Disabilities*. New York: Guilford Press.

Emerson, E. and Glover, G. (2011). *Health Checks for People with Learning Disabilities: 2008/9–2010/11*. Durham: Improving Health and Lives: Learning Disabilities Observatory.

Emerson, E. and Glover, G. (2012). The 'transition cliff' in the administrative prevalence of learning disabilities in England. *Tizard Learning Disability Review*, 17, 139–43.

Emerson, E., Graham, H. and Hatton, C. (2006a). Household income and health status in children and adolescents: Cross-sectional study. *European Journal of Public Health*, 16, 354–60.

Emerson, E., Graham, H. and Hatton, C. (2006b). The measurement of poverty and socio-economic position in research involving people with intellectual disability. In L. M. Glidden (ed.), *International Review of Research in Mental Retardation*. New York: Academic Press, pp. 77–108.

Emerson, E. and Halpin, S. (2013). Anti-social behaviour and police contact among 13–15-year-old English adolescents with and without mild/moderate intellectual disability. *Journal of Applied Research in Intellectual Disabilities*, 26, 362–9.

Emerson, E. and Hatton, C. (2007a). The contribution of socio-economic position to the health inequalities faced by children and adolescents with intellectual disabilities in Britain. *American Journal on Mental Retardation*, 112, 140–50.

Emerson, E. and Hatton, C. (2007b). The mental health of children and adolescents with intellectual disabilities in Britain. *British Journal of Psychiatry*, 191, 493–9.

Emerson, E. and Hatton, C. (2007c). Poverty, socio-economic position, social capital and the health of children and adolescents with intellectual disabilities in Britain: A replication. *Journal of Intellectual Disability Research*, 51, 866–74.

Emerson, E. and Hatton, C. (2008a). *People with Learning Disabilities in England*. Lancaster: Centre for Disability Research, Lancaster University.

Emerson, E. and Hatton, C. (2008b). The self-reported well-being of women and men with intellectual disabilities in England. *American Journal on Mental Retardation*, 113, 143–55.

Emerson, E. and Hatton, C. (2008c). Socio-economic disadvantage, social participation and networks, and the self-rated health of English men and women with mild and moderate intellectual disabilities: Cross-sectional survey. *European Journal of Public Health*, 18, 31–7.

Emerson, E. and Hatton, C. (2010). Socio-economic position, poverty and family research. In L. M. Glidden and M. M. Seltzer (eds.), *On Families: International Review of Research on Mental Retardation*. New York: Academic Press.

Emerson, E. and Hatton, C. (2011). *Estimating Future Need for Adult Social Care Services for People with Learning Disabilities in England: An Update*. Stockton-on-Tees: Learning Disabilities Public Health Observatory, North East Public Health Observatory.

Emerson, E., Hatton, C., Hastings, R. et al. (2011c). The health of people with autistic spectrum disorders. *Tizard Learning Disability Review*, 16(4), 36–45.

Emerson, E., Hatton, C. and Robertson, J. (2011d). *Prevention and Social Care for Adults with Learning Disabilities*. London: NIHR School for Social Care Research.

Emerson, E., Hatton, C., Robertson, J. et al. (2011e). *People with Learning Disabilities in England: 2010*. Durham: Improving Health and Lives: Learning Disabilities Observatory.

Emerson, E., Hatton, C., Robertson, J. et al. (2012b). *People with Learning Disabilities in England: 2011*. Durham: Improving Health and Lives: Learning Disabilities Observatory.

Emerson, E., Hatton, C., Robertson, J. et al. (2013). *People with Learning Disabilities in England: 2012*. Durham: Improving Health and Lives: Learning Disabilities Observatory.

Emerson, E. and Jahoda, A. J. (2013). Social and psychological factors as determinants of emotional and behavioural difficulties. In J. L. Taylor, W. R. Lindsay, R. P. Hastings and C. Hatton (eds.), *Psychological Therapies for Adults with Intellectual Disabilities*. Chichester: Wiley-Blackwell, pp. 15–30.

Emerson, E., Kiernan, C., Alborz, A. et al. (2001). The prevalence of challenging behaviors: A total population study. *Research in Developmental Disabilities*, 22, 77–93.

Emerson, E., Madden, R., Graham, H. et al. (2011f). The health of disabled people and the social determinants of health. *Public Health*, 125, 145–7.

Emerson, E., Madden, R., Robertson, J. et al. (2009). *Intellectual and Physical Disability, Social Mobility, Social Inclusion and Health: Background Paper for the Marmot Review*. Lancaster: Centre for Disability Research, Lancaster University.

Emerson, E., Malam, S., Davies, I. and Spencer, K. (2005). *Adults with Learning Difficulties in England 2003/4*. Leeds: Health and Social Care Information Centre.

Emerson, E., McCulloch, A., Graham, H. et al. (2010). The mental health of parents of young children with and without developmental delays. *American Journal on Intellectual and Developmental Disability*, 115, 30–42.

Emerson, E. and McVilly, K. (2004). Friendship activities of adults with intellectual disabilities in supported accommodation in Northern England. *Journal of Applied Research in Intellectual Disabilities*, 17, 191–7.

Emerson, E. and Robertson, J. (2008). *Commissioning Person-centred, Cost-effective, Local Support for People with Learning Difficulties*. London: SCIE.

Emerson, E. and Robertson, J. (2010). Obesity in young children with intellectual disabilities or borderline intellectual functioning. *International Journal of Pediatric Obesity*, 5(4), 320–6.

Emerson, E. and Robertson, J. (2011). *The Estimated Prevalence of Visual Impairment among People with Learning Disabilities in England: Improving Health and Lives*. Cambridge: Learning Disabilities Observatory.

Emerson, E., Robertson, J., Gregory, N. et al. (2000). The treatment and management of challenging behaviours in residential settings. *Journal of Applied Research in Intellectual Disabilities*, 13, 197–215.

Emerson, E. and Roulstone, A. (in press). Developing an evidence base for violent and disablist hate crime in the Britain: Findings from the Life Opportunities Survey. *Journal of Interpersonal Violence*.

Emerson, E., Shahtahmasebi, S., Lancaster, G. and Berridge, D. (2010). Poverty transitions among families supporting a child with intellectual disability. *Journal of Intellectual and Developmental Disability*, 35(4), 224–34.

Emerson, E. and Turnbull, L. (2005). Self-reported smoking and alcohol use by adolescents with and without intellectual disabilities. *Journal of Intellectual Disabilities*, 9, 58–69.

Emerson, E., Vick, B., Graham, H. et al. (2012c). Disablement and health. In N. Watson, C. Thomas and A. Roulstone (eds.), *Routledge Companion to Disability Studies*. London: Routledge.

Emerson, E., Vick, B., Rechel, B. et al. (In press). *Health Inequalities and People with Disabilities in Europe*. Copenhagen: European Regional Office of the World Health Organization.

Engels, F. (1969). *The Condition of the Working Class in England: From Personal Observation and Authentic Sources (first published 1845, Leipzig)*. London: Granada Press.

Esbensen, A. J. and Benson, B. A. (2006). A prospective analysis of life events, problem behaviours and depression in adults with intellectual disability. *Journal of Intellectual Disability Research*, 50, 248–58.

Evenhuis, H. M. (2001). Prevalence of visual and hearing impairment in a Dutch institutionalized population with intellectual disability. *Journal of Intellectual Disability Research*, 45, 457–64.

Evenhuis, H. M., Hermans, H., Hilgenkamp, T. I. M., Bastiaanse, L. P. and Echteld, M. A. (2012). Frailty and disability in older adults with intellectual disabilities: Results from the Healthy Ageing and Intellectual Disability Study. *Journal of the American Geriatrics Society*, 60, 934–8.

Faulks, D. and Hennequin, M. (2000). Evaluation of a long-term oral health program by carers of children and adults with intellectual disabilities. *Special Care in Dentistry*, 20(5), 10.

Fedele, S. and Scully, C. (2010). Dentition and oral health diseases. In J. O'Hara, J. E. McCarthy and N. Bouras (eds.), *Intellectual Disability and Ill Health: A Review of the Evidence*. Cambridge University Press, pp. 151–61.

Felce, D., Baxter, H., Lowe, K. et al. (2008a). The impact of repeated health checks for adults with intellectual disabilities. *Journal of Applied Research in Intellectual Disabilities*, 21(6), 585–96. DOI: 10.1111/j.1468-3148.2008.00441.x.

Felce, D., Baxter, H., Lowe, K. et al. (2008b). The impact of checking the health of adults with intellectual disabilities on primary care consultation rates, health promotion and contact with specialists. *Journal of Applied Research in Intellectual Disabilities*, 21, 597–602.

Fernandez, J. B., Lim, L. J., Dougherty, N. et al. (2012). Oral health findings in athletes with intellectual disabilities at the NYC Special Olympics. *Special Care Dentistry*, 32, 205–9.

Ferrari, M. (2009). Borderline intellectual functioning and the intellectual disability construct. *Intellectual and Developmental Disabilities*, 47, 386–9.

Ferri, M. A., Amato, L. and Davoli, M. (2006). Alcoholics Anonymous and other 12-step programmes for alcohol dependence. *Cochrane Database of Systematic Reviews*, CD005032.

Fickert, N. A. and Ross, D. (2012). Effectiveness of a caregiver education program on providing oral care to individuals with intellectual and developmental disabilities. *Intellectual and Developmental Disabilities,* 50(3), 14.

Fidler, W., Michell, R. G. and Charlton, A. (1992). Smoking: A special need? *British Journal of Addiction*, 87, 1583–91.

Finlay, W. M. L. and Lyons, E. (2001). Methodological issues in interviewing and using self-report questionnaires with people with mental retardation. *Psychological Assessment*, 13, 319–35.

Finlayson, J., Morrison, J., Jackson, A., Mantry, D. and Cooper, S. A. (2010). Injuries, falls and accidents among adults with intellectual disabilities. Prospective cohort study. *Journal of Intellectual Disability Research*, 54, 966–80.

Fischer, L. S., Becker, A., Paraguya, M., Chukwa, C. (2012). Colonoscopy and colorectal cancer screening in adults with intellectual and developmental disabilities: Review of a series of cases and recommendations for examination. *Intellectual and Developmental Disabilities,* 50(5), 8.

Fisher, K. (2004). Health disparities and mental retardation. *Journal of Nursing Scholarship*, 36, 48–53.

Fleming, R.K., Stokes, E.A., Curtin, C., Bandini, L.G., Gleason, J., Scampini, R., Maslin, M.C.T., Hamad, C. (2008). Behavioral health in developmental disabilities: A comprehensive program of nutrition, exercise, and weight reduction. *International Journal of Behavioral Consultation and Therapy*, 4(3), 10.

Flynn, J. R. (1987). Massive Iq gains in 14 nations – what IQ tests really measure. *Psychological Bulletin*, 101(2), 171–91.

Forrester-Jones, R., Carpenter, J., Coolen-Schrinjer, P. et al. (2006). The social networks of people with intellectual disability living in the community 12 years after resettlement from long-stay hospitals. *Journal of Applied Research in Intellectual Disabilities*, 19, 285–95.

Fossett, B. and Mirenda, P. (2007). Augmentative and alternative communication. In S. L. Odom, R. Horner, M. E. Snell and J. Blacher (eds.), *Handbook of Developmental Disabilities*. New York: Guilford.

Foster, C. H., Hillsdon, M., Thorogood, M., Kaur, A., and Wedatilake, T. (2005). Interventions for promoting physical activity. *Cochrane Database of Systematic Reviews*, CD003180.

Fowler, P. J., Tompsett, C. J., Braciszewski, J. B., Jacques-Tiura, A. J. and Baltes, B. B. (2009). Community violence: A meta-analysis on the effect of exposure and mental health outcomes of children and adolescents. *Development and Psychopathology*, 21 227–59.

Foxcroft, D. R. T. and Tsertsvadze, A. (2011). Universal family-based prevention programs for alcohol misuse in young people. *Cochrane Database of Systematic Reviews*, CD009308.

Fraser, S. and Sim, J. (2007). *The Sexual Health Needs of Young People with Learning Disabilities*. Edinburgh: Health Scotland.

Frieden, T. R. (2010). A framework for public health action: The health impact pyramid. *American Journal of Public Health*, 100(4), 6.

Fryers, T. (1993). Epidemiological thinking in mental retardation: Issues in taxonomy and population frequency. In N. W. Bray (ed.), *International Review of Research in Mental Retardation, Vol. 19*. San Diego, CA: Academic Press.

Fujiura, G. T. (1998). Demography of family households. *American Journal on Mental Retardation*, 103, 225–35.

Fujiura, G. T. (2012). Self-reported health of people with intellectual disability. *Intellectual and Developmental Disabilities*, 50, 352–69.

Gardiner, T. and Braddon, E. (2009). 'A right to know': facilitating a relationship and sexuality programme for adults with intellectual disabilities in Donegal. *British Journal of Learning Disabilities*, 37, 3.

Gebel, K., Bauman, A. E. and Bull, F. C. (2010). Built environment: Walkability of neighbourhoods. In A. Killoran and M. P. Kelly (eds.), *Evidence-based Public Health: Effectiveness and Efficiency*. Oxford University Press, pp. 298–312.

Gee, G. C., Ro, A., Shariff-Marco, S. and Chae, D. (2009). Racial discrimination and health among Asian Americans: Evidence, assessment, and directions for future research. *Epidemiologic Reviews*, 31, 130–51.

Gibson, P. A., Newton, R. W., Selby, K. et al. (2005). Longitudinal study of thyroid function in Down's syndrome in the first two decades. *Archive of Diseases of Childhood*, 90, 574–8.

Gilbert, R., Widom, C. S., Browne, K. et al. (2009). Burden and consequences of child maltreatment in high-income countries. *Lancet*, 373, 68–81.

Gilbert-McLeod, C. A., Craig, K. D., Rocha, E. M. and Mathias, M. D. (2000). Everyday pain responses in children with and without developmental delays. *Journal of Pediatric Psychology*, 25, 301–8.

Gillam, S., Yates, J. and Badrinath, P. (eds.). (2007). *Essential Public Health*. Cambridge University Press.

Giraud-Saunders, A. (2009). *Equal Access? A Practical Guide for the NHS: Creating a Single Equality Scheme that Includes Improving Access for People with Learning Disabilities*. London: Department of Health.

Glaser, D. (2008). Child sexual abuse. In M. Rutter, D. Bishop, D. Pine, S. Scott, J. Stevenson, E. Taylor and A. Thapar (eds.), *Rutter's Child and Adolescent Psychiatry*. Oxford: Blackwell, pp. 440–58.

Glover, G. and Ayub, M. (2010). *How People with Learning Disabilities Die*. Durham: Improving Health and Lives: Learning Disabilities Observatory.

Glover, G. and Emerson, E. (2012a). *Have You Got a Learning Disability? Asking the Question and Recording the Answer for NHS Healthcare Providers*. Durham: Improving Health and Lives: Learning Disabilities Public Health Observatory.

Glover, G.; Emerson, E.; Baines, S. (2011). *NHS data gaps for learning disabilities: The information the NHS needs to monitor the health and healthcare of people with learning disabilities*. Durham: Learning Disabilities Public Health Observatory.

Glover, G. and Emerson, E. (2012b). Patterns of decline in numbers of learning disability nurses employed by the English National Health Service. *Tizard Learning Disability Review*, 17, 194–8.

Glover, G., Emerson, E. and Eccles, R. (2012a). *Using Local Data to Monitor the Health Needs of People with Learning Disabilities*. Durham: Improving Health and Lives: Learning Disabilities Public Health Observatory.

Glover, G., Emerson, E. and Evison, F. (2012b). *The Uptake of Health Checks for Adults with Learning Disabilities: 2008/9 to 2011/12*. Durham: Improving Health and Lives: Learning Disabilities Public Health Observatory.

Glover, G., Emerson, E. and Evison, F. (2013). The uptake of annnual health checks for adults with learning disabilities in England: 2008/9 to 2011/12. *Tizard Learning Disability Review*, 18, 45–9.

Glover, G. and Evison, F. (2013). *Hospital Admissions That Should Not Happen: Admissions for Ambulatory Care-Sensitive Conditions for People with Learning Disabilities in England*. Stockton-on-Tees: Learning Disabilities Public Health Observatory.

Glover, G. and Olson, V. (2012). *Assessment and Treatment Units and Other Specialist Inpatient Care for People with Learning Disabilities in the Count-Me-In Surveys, 2006 to 2010*. Durham: Learning Disabilities Public Health Observatory.

Golubovic, S. M., Maksimovic, J., Golubovic, B. and Glumbic, N. (2012). Effects of exercise on physical fitness in children with intellectual disability. *Research in Developmental Disabilities*, 33, 7.

Government Equalities Office. (2010). *Equality Act 2010: What Do I Need to Know? Disability Quick Start Guide*. London: Government Equalities Office.

Graham, H. (2005). Intellectual disabilities and socio-economic inequalities in health: An overview of research. *Journal of Applied Research in Intellectual Disabilities*, 18, 101–11.

Graham, H. (2007). *Unequal Lives: Health and Socio-economic Inequalities*. Maidenhead: Open University Press.

Graham, H. and Power, C. (2010). Equity, risk, and the life-course: A framework for understanding and tackling health inequalities. In A. Killoran and M. P. Kelly (eds.), *Evidence-based Public Health: Effectiveness and Efficiency*. Oxford University Press, pp. 63–78.

Grant, H. J., Pickett, W., Lam, M., O'Connor, M. and Ouellette-Kuntz, H. (2001). Falls among persons who have developmental disabilities in institutional and group home settings. *Journal on Developmental Disabilities*, 8, 57–73.

Grantham-McGregor, S., Cheung, Y. B., Cueto, S. et al. (2007). Developmental potential in the first 5 years for children in developing countries. *Lancet*, 369, 60–70.

Gray, K., Keating, C., Taffe, J. et al. (2012). Trajectory of behavior and emotional problems in autism. *American Journal on Intellectual and Developmental Disabilities*, 117, 121–33.

Green, S. E. (2007). 'We're tired, not sad': Benefits and burdens of mothering a child with a disability. *Social Science and Medicine*, 64, 150–63.

Grosse, S. D., Lollar, D. J., Campbell, V. A. and Chamie, M. (2009). Disability and disability-adjusted life years: Not the same. *Public Health Reports*, 124, 197–202.

Hahn, J. E. and Aronow, H. U. (2005). A pilot of a gerontological advanced practice nurse preventive intervention. *Journal of Applied Research in Intellectual Disabilities*, 18(2), 131–42.

Hamilton, D., Sutherland, G. and Iacono, T. (2005). Further examination of relationships between life events and psychiatric symptoms in adults with intellectual disability. *Journal of Intellectual Disability Research*, 49, 839–44.

Hanna, L. M., Taggart, L. and Cousins, W. (2011). Cancer prevention and health promotion for people with intellectual disabilities: An exploratory study of staff knowledge. *Journal of Intellectual Disability Research*, 55, 281–91.

Harden, A., Brunton, G., Fletcher, A. *et al.* (2006). *Young People, Pregnancy and Social Exclusion: A Systematic Synthesis of Research Evidence to Identify Effective, Appropriate and Promising Approaches for Prevention and Support*. London: EPPI-Centre, Social Science Research Unit, Institute of Education, University of London.

Harding, C. and Wright, J. (2010). Dysphagia: The challenge of managing eating and drinking difficulties in children and adults who have learning disabilities. *Tizard Learning Disability Review*, 15, 4–13.

Harrell, E. (2011). Disability and victimization in a national sample of children and youth. *Child Maltreatment*, 16, 275–86.

Harrell, E. (2012). *Crime against People with Disabilities, 2009–2011 Statistical Tables*. http://bjs.gov/content/pub/pdf/capd0911st.pdf. Washington: US Department of Justice.

Harris, J. C. (2005). *Intellectual Disability: Understanding Its Development, Causes, Evaluation, and Treatment*. Oxford University Press.

Hartley, S. and MacLean, W. (2006). A review of the reliability and validity of Likert-type scales for people with intellectual disabilities. *Journal of Intellectual Disabilities Research*, 50, 813–27.

Hasle, H., Clemmensen, I. H. and Mikkelsen, M. (2000). Risks of leukaemia and solid tumours in individuals with Down's syndrome. *Lancet*, 355, 165–9.

Hassiotis, A., Barron, P. and O'Hara, J. (2000). Mental health services for people with learning disabilities: A complete overhaul is needed with strong links to mainstream services. *British Medical Journal*, 321, 583–4.

Hassiotis, A., Strydom, A., Hall, I. et al. (2008). Psychiatric morbidity and social functioning among adults with borderline intelligence living in private households. *Journal of Intellectual Disability Research*, 52(2), 95–106.

Hastings, R. P. (2007). Longitudinal relationships between sibling behavioral adjustment and behavior problems of children with developmental disabilities. *Journal of Autism and Developmental Disorders*, 37, 1485–92.

Hastings, R. P., Hatton, C., Taylor, J. L. and Maddison, C. (2004). Life events and psychiatric symptoms in adults with intellectual disabilities. *Journal of Intellectual Disability Research* 48, 42–6.

Hatton, C. (1998). Whose quality of life is it anyway? Some problems with the emerging quality of life consensus. *Mental Retardation*, 36, 104–15.

Hatton, C. (2002). People with intellectual disabilities from ethnic minority communities in the United States and the United Kingdom. *International Review of Research in Mental Retardation*, 25, 209–39.

Hatton, C., Akram, Y., Robertson, J., Shah, R. and Emerson, E. (2003). *Supporting South Asian Families with a Child with Severe Disabilities*. London: Jessica Kingsley.

Hatton, C., Azmi, S., Caine, A. and Emerson, E. (1998). People from the South Asian communities who care for adolescents and adults with intellectual disabilities: Family circumstances, service support and carer stress. *British Journal of Social Work*, 28, 821–37.

Hatton, C., Roberts, H. and Baines, S. (2011). *Reasonable Adjustments for People with Learning Disabilities in England: A National Survey of NHS Trusts.* Durham: North East Public Health Observatory.

Hatton, C. and Taylor, J. L. (2013). The assessment of mental health problems in adults with intellectual disabilities. In J. L. Taylor, W. R. Lindsay, R. P. Hastings and C. Hatto (eds.), *Psychological Therapies for Adults with Intellectual Disabilities.* Chichester: Wiley-Blackwell, pp. 31–54.

Hauland, H. and Allen, C. (2009). *Deaf People and Human Rights.* Helsinki: World Federation of the Deaf.

Haveman, M., Heller, T., Lee, L. et al. (2010). Major health risks in aging persons with intellectual disabilities: An overview of recent studies. *Journal of Policy and Practice in Intellectual Disabilities*, 7, 59–69.

Havercamp, S., Scandlin, D. and Roth, M. (2004). Health disparities among adults with developmental disabilities, adults with other disabilities, and adults not reporting disability in North Carolina. *Public Health Reports*, 119, 9.

Hawkins, A. and Look, R. (2006). Levels of engagement and barriers to physical activity in a population of adults with learning disabilities. *British Journal of Learning Disabilities*, 34, 220–6.

Headey, B. and Wearing, A. (1989). Personality, life events and subjective well-being: Toward a dynamic equilibrium model. *Journal of Personality and Social Psychology*, 57, 731–9.

Heber, R. (1970). *Epidemiology of Mental Retardation.* Springfield, IL: Charles C. Thomas.

Heller, T. M., McCubbin, J.-A., Drum, C. and Peterson, J. (2011). Physical activity and nutrition health promotion interventions: What is working for people with intellectual disabilities? *Intellectual and Developmental Disabilities*, 49(1), 11.

Heloma, A., Jaakkola, M. S., Kahkonen, E. and Reijula, K. (2001). The short-term impact of national smoke-free workplace legislation on passive smoking and tobacco use. *American Journal of Public Health*, 91, 1416–18.

Henderson, C., Evans-Lacko, S. and Thornicroft, G. (2013). Mental illness stigmas, help seeking, and public health programs. *American Journal of Public Health*, 103, 777–80.

Hermon, C., Alberman, E., Beral, V. and Swerdlow, A. J. (2001). Mortality and cancer incidence in persons with Down's syndrome, their parents and siblings. *Annals of Human Genetics*, 65, 167–76.

Hertzman, C. and Boyce, T. (2010). How experience gets under the skin to create gradients in developmental health. *Annual Review of Public Health*, 31, 329–47.

Heslop, P., Blair, P., Fleming, P. et al. (2013). *Confidential Inquiry Into Premature Deaths of People with Learning Disabilities.* Bristol: Norah Fry Research Centre.

Hipp, J. R. and Lakon, C. M. (2010). Social disparities in health: Disproportionate toxicity proximity in minority communities over a decade. *Health and Place*, 16, 674–83.

Hoeve, M., Dubas, J. S., Eichelsheim, V. I. et al. (2009). The relationship between parenting and delinquency: A meta-analysis. *Journal of Abnormal Child Psychology*, 37, 749–75.

Hogg, J. and Tuffrey-Wijne, I. (2009). Cancer and intellectual disability: A review of some key contextual issues. *Journal of Applied Research in Intellectual Disabilities*, 21, 509–18.

Holden, B. and Gitlesen, J. P. (2006). A total population study of challenging behaviour in the county of Hedmark, Norway: Prevalence and risk markers. *Research in Developmental Disabilities*, 27, 456–65.

Holland, A. J., Hon, J., Huppert, F. A., Stevens, S. and Watson, P. (1998). Population-based study of the prevalence and presentation of dementia in adults with Down's syndrome. *British Journal of Psychiatry*, 172, 493–8.

Hollins, S., Attard, M., van Fraunhofer, N., McGuigan, S. M. and Sedgwick, P. (1998). Mortality in people with learning disability: Risks, causes and death certification findings in London. *Developmental Medicine and Child Neurology*, 40, 50–6.

House, J. S., Landis, K. R. and Umberson, D. (1988). Social relationships and health. *Science*, 241, 540–5.

House of Lords and House of Commons Joint Committee on Human Rights. (2008). *A Life Like Any Other? Human Rights of Adults with Learning Disabilities*. London: The Stationery Office Limited.

Howe, T. (2010). *Life Opportunities Survey: Interim Results 2009/10*. London: Office for National Statistics.

Hsieh, K., Heller, T. and Miller, A. B. (2001). Risk factors for injuries and falls among adults with developmental disabilities. *Journal of Intellectual Disability Research*, 45, 76–82.

Hsieh, K., Rimmer, J. and Heller, T. (2012). Prevalence of falls and risk factors in adults with intellectual disability. *American Journal on Intellectual and Developmental Disability*, 117, 442–54.

Hsu, S., Lin, J., Chiang, P., Chang, Y. and Tung, H. (2012a). Comparison of outpatient services between elderly people with intellectual disabilities and the general elderly population in Taiwan. *Research in Developmental Disabilities*, 33, 1429–36.

Hsu, S., Yen, C., Hung, W. et al. (2012b). The risk of metabolic syndrome among institutionalized adults with intellectual disabilities. *Research in Developmental Disabilities*, 33, 615–20.

Hsu, S., Yen, C., Hung, W. et al. (2012c). The risk of metabolic syndrome among institutionalized adults with intellectual disabilities. *Research in Developmental Disabilities*, 33, 615–20.

Hughes, K., Bellis, M. A., Jones, L. et al. (2012). Prevalence and risk of violence against adults with disabilities: A systematic review and meta-analysis of observational studies. *Lancet*, 379(9826), 1621–9.

Hulbert-Williams, L. and Hastings, R. P. (2008). Life events as a risk factor for psychological problems in individuals with intellectual disabilities: A critical review. *Journal of Intellectual Disability Research*, 52, 883–95.

Humphries, K., Pepper, A., Traci, M. A., Olson, J. and Seekins, T. (2009a). Nutritional intervention improves menu adequacy in group homes for adults with intellectual or developmental disabilities. *Disability and Health Journal*, 2, 136–44.

Humphries, K., Traci, M. A. and Seekins, T. (2009b). Nutrition and adults with intellectual or developmental disabilities: Systematic literature review results. *Intellectual and Developmental Disabilities*, 47, 163–85.

IASSID Special Interest Research Group on Parents and Parenting with Intellectual Disabilities. (2008). Parents labelled with intellectual disability: Position of the IASSID SIRG on Parents and Parenting with Intellectual Disabilities. *Journal of Applied Research in Intellectual Disabilities*, 21, 296–307.

Idler, E. L. and Benyamini, Y. (1997). Self-rated health and mortality: A review of twenty-seven community studies. *Journal of Health and Social Behavior*, 38, 21–37.

Idler, E. L. and Benyamini, Y. (1999). Community studies reporting association between self-rated health and mortality: Additional studies, 1995 to 1998. *Research on Aging*, 21, 392–401.

Institute of Medicine. (2001). *Neurological, Psychiatric, and Developmental Disorders: Meeting the Challenge in the Developing World*. Washington DC: National Academy Press.

IoM. (1988). *The Future of Public Health*. Washington DC.

Irish, L., Kobayashi, I. and Delahanty, D. L. (2010). Long-term physical health consequences of childhood sexual abuse: A meta-analytic review. *Journal of Pediatric Psychology*, 35, 450–61.

Irving, C. A. and Chaudhari, M.P. (2012). Cardiovascular abnormalities in Down's syndrome: spectrum, management and survival over 22 years. *Archives of Disease in Childhood*, 97(4), 5.

Irwin, L. G., Siddiqi, A. and Hertzman, C. (2007). *Early Child Development: A Powerful Equalizer*. Geneva: World Health Organization.

Iyer, A. (2007). Depiction of intellectual disability in fiction. *Advances in Psychiatric Treatment*, 13, 127–33.

Jacobson, C., Shearer, J., Habel, A. et al. (2010). Core neuropsychological characteristics of children and adolescents with 22q11.2 deletion. *Journal of Intellectual Disability Research*, 54, 701–13.

Jaffe, J. S., Timell, A. M., Elolia, R. and Thatcher, S. S. (2005). Risk factors for low bone mineral density in individuals residing in a facility for people with intellectual disability. *Journal of Intellectual Disability Research*, 49, 457–62.

Jaffe, J. S., Timell, A. M. and Gulanski, B. I. (2001). Prevalence of low bone density in women with developmental disabilities. *Journal of Clinical Densitometry*, 4, 25–9.

Jancar, J. (1990). Cancer and mental handicap: A further study. *British Journal of Psychiatry*, 156, 531–3.

Janicki, M. P., Davidson, P. W., Henderson, C. M. et al. (2002). Health characteristics and health services utilization in older adults with intellectual disability living in community residences. *Journal of Intellectual Disability Research*, 46, 287–98.

Jansen, J., Rozeboom, W., Penning, C. and Evenhuis, H. M. (2013). Prevalence and incidence of myocardial infarction and cerebrovascular accident in ageing persons with intellectual disability. *Journal of Intellectual Disability Reasearch*, 57(7), 681–5.

Jenkins, J. (2008). Psychosocial adversity and resilience. In M. Rutter, D. Bishop, D. Pine, S. Scott, J. Stevenson, E. Taylor and A. Thapar (eds.), *Rutter's Child and Adolescent Psychiatry* (5th edn). Oxford: Blackwell, pp. 377–91.

Jenkins, R. (1998). *Questions of Competence: Culture, Classification and Intellectual Disability*. Cambridge University Press.

Jensen, K. M. and Davis, M. M. (2013). Healthcare in adults with Down syndrome: A longitudinal cohort study. *Journal of Intellectual Disabilities Research*, 57(5), 409–21.

Jensen, K. M., Taylor, L. C. and Davis, M. M. (in press). Primary care for adults with Down syndrome: adherence to preventive healthcare recommendations.

Jobling, A. and Cuskelly, M. (2006). Young people with Down syndrome: A preliminary investigation of health knowledge and associated behaviours. *Journal of Intellectual and Developmental Disability*, 31, 210–18.

Jones, D. P. H. (2008). Child maltreatment. In M. Rutter, D. Bishop, D. Pine, S. Scott, J. Stevenson, E. Taylor and A. Thapar (eds.), *Rutter's Child and Adolescent Psychiatry*. Oxford: Blackwell, pp. 421–39.

Jones, J., Hathaway, D., Gilhooley, M., Leech, A. and MacLeod, S. (2010). Down syndrome health screening – the Fife model. *British Journal of Learning Disabilities*, 38, 5–9.

Jones, L., Bellis, M. A., Wood, S. et al. (2012). Prevalence and risk of violence against children with disabilities: A systematic review and meta-analysis of observational studies. *Lancet*, 380(9845), 899–907.

Jones, R. G. and Kerr, M. P. (1997). A randomized control trial of an opportunistic health screening tool in primary care for people with intellectual disability. [Proceedings Paper.] *Journal of Intellectual Disability Research*, 41, 409–15.

Jylha, M. (2009). What is self-rated health and why does it predict mortality? Towards a unified conceptual model. *Social Science and Medicine*, 69, 307–16.

Kahneman, D., Diener, E. and Schwarz, N. (eds.). (1999). *Well-Being: The Foundations of Hedonic Psychology*. New York: Russel Sage Foundation.

Kaiser, A. P. and Trent, J. A. (2007). Communication intervention for young children with disabilities. In S. L. Odom, R. Horner, M. E. Snell and J. Blacher (eds.), *Handbook of Developmental Disabilities*. New York: Guilford.

Kaner, E. F., Beyer, F., Dickinson, H.-O. et al. (2007). Effectiveness of brief alcohol interventions in primary care populations. *Cochrane Database of Systematic Reviews*, CD 004148.

Kannabiran, M. and Deb, S. (2010). Diseases of the nervous system I: Neurodegenerative diseases including dementias. In J. O'Hara, J. E. McCarthy and N. Bouras (eds.), *Intellectual Disability and Ill Health: A Review of the Evidence*. Cambridge University Press, pp. 203–13.

Katusic, S. A., Colligan, R. C., Beard, M. et al. (1995). Mental retardation in a birth cohort, 1976–1980, Rochester, Minnesota. *American Journal on Mental Retardation*, 100, 335–44.

Kawachi, I. and Berkman, L. F. (2000). Social cohesion, social capital, and health. In L. F. Berkman and I. Kawachi (eds.), *Social Epidemiology*. New York: Oxford University Press, pp. 174–90.

Kawachi, I. and Berkman, L. F. (eds.). (2003). *Neighborhoods and Health*. Oxford University Press.

Kerker, B. D., Owens, P. L., Zigler, E. and Horwitz, S. M. (2004). Mental health disorders among individuals with mental retardation: Challenges to accurate prevalence estimates. *Public Health Reports*, 119(4), 409–17.

Kerr, A. M., McCulloch, D., Oliver, K. et al. (2003). Medical needs of people with intellectual disability require regular reassessment, and the provision of client- and carer-held reports. *Journal of Intellectual Disability Research*, 47, 134–45.

Kerr, M. and Bowley, C. (2001a). Evidence-based prescribing in adults with learning disability and epilepsy. *Epilepsia*, 42(Suppl. 1), 44–5.

Kerr, M. and Bowley, C. (2001b). Multidisciplinary and multiagency contributions to care for those with learning disability who have epilepsy. *Epilepsia*, 42(Suppl. 1), 55–6.

Kerr, M., Felce, D. and Felce, J. (2005). *Equal Treatment: Closing the Gap. Final Report from the Welsh Centre for Learning Disabilities to the Disability Rights Commission*. Cardiff: Welsh Centre for Learning Disabilities, Cardiff University.

Kerr, M. P., Richards, D. and Glover, G. (1996). Primary care for people with a learning disability – a Group Practice survey. *Journal of Applied Research in Intellectual Disability*, 9, 347–52.

Kiely, M. (1987). The prevalence of mental retardation. *Epidemiologic Reviews*, 9, 194–218.

Kiernan, C., Reeves, D. and Alborz, A. (1995). The use of anti-psychotic drugs with adults with learning disabilities and challenging behaviour. *Journal of Intellectual Disability Research*, 39, 263–74.

Killoran, A. and Kelly, M. P. (eds.). (2010). *Evidence-based Public Health: Effectiveness and Efficiency.* Oxford University Press.

Killoran, A. O. and Bauld, L. (2006). Smoking cessation: An evidence-based approach to tackling health inequalities? In A. S. Killoran and C. Kelly (eds.), *Public Health Evidence: Tackling Health Inequalities.* Oxford University Press, pp. 341–62.

Klenerman, P., Sander, J. W. and Shorvon, S. D. (1993). Mortality in patients with epilepsy: A study of patients in long-term residential care. *Journal Of Neurology, Neurosurgery and Psychiatry*, 56(2), 149–52.

Knapp, W. P. S., Soares, B., Farrell, M. and Silva de Lima, M. (2007). Psychosocial interventions for cocaine- and psychostimulant amphetamines-related disorders. *Cochrane Database of Systematic Reviews*, CD003023.

Krahn, G. and Campbell, V. A. (2011). Evolving views of disability and public health: The roles of advocacy and public health. *Disability and Health Journal*, 4, 7.

Krahn, G. and Fox, M. H. (In press). Health disparities of adults with intellectual disabilities: What do we know? What do we do? *Journal of Applied Research in Intellectual Disability.*

Krahn, G., Fox, M. H., Campbell, V. A., Ramon, I. and Jesien, G. (2010). Developing a health surveillance system for people with intellectual disabilities in the United States. *Journal of Policy and Practice in Intellectual Disabilities*, 7, 155–66.

Krahn, G. L., Hammond, L. and Turner, A. (2006). A cascade of disparities: Health and healthcare access for people with intellectual disabilities. *Mental Retardation and Developmental Disabilities Research Reviews*, 12, 70–82.

Kreiger, N. (2011). *Epidemiology and the People's Health: Theory and Context.* Oxford University Press.

Krieger, N. (1999). Embodying inequality: A review of concepts, measures, and methods for studying health consequences of discrimination. *International Journal of Health Services*, 29, 295–352.

Kwok, H. and Cheung, P. W. H. (2007). Co-morbidity of psychiatric disorder and medical illness in people with intellectual disabilities. *Current Opinion in Psychiatry*, 20, 443–9.

Lagu, T., Hannon, N. S., Rothberg, M. B. et al. (2013). Access to subspecialty care for patients with mobility impairment: A survey. *Annals of Internal Medicine*, 158, 441–6.

Lancaster, T. S. and Stead, L.-F. (2008). Individual behavioural counselling for smoking cessation. *Cochrane Database of Systematic Reviews*, CD001292.

Larson, S., Lakin, C., Anderson, L. and Kwak, N. (2001a). *Characteristics of and Service Use by Persons with MR/DD Living in Their Own Homes or With Family Members: NHIS-D Analysis.* Minneapolis, MN: Research and Training Center on Community Living, Institute on Community Integration, University of Minnesota.

Larson, S., Lakin, K. C., Anderson, L. et al. (2001b). Prevalence of mental retardation and developmental disabilities: Estimates from the 1994/1995 National Health Interview Survey Disability Supplements. *American Journal on Mental Retardation*, 106, 231–52.

Larson, S., Lakin, K. C. and Anderson, L. L. (2003). Definitions and findings on intellectual and developmental disabilities within the NHIS-D. In B. M. Altman, S. N. Barnartt, G. E. Hendershot and S. A. Larson (eds.), *Using Survey Data to Study Disability: Results from the National Health Interview Survey on Disability.* Boston, MA: Elsevier, pp. 229–55.

Larson, S. L., Lakin, C.-L. and Huang, J. (2003). Service use by and needs of adults with functional limitations or ID/DD in the NHS-D: Difference by age, gender, and disability. *DD Data Brief*, 5(2), 25.

Lau, J. T.-F. and Cheung, C.-K. (1999). Discriminatory attitudes to people with intellectual disability or mental health difficulty. *International Social Work*, 42, 431–44.

Lauer, E. (2010). *2008 Mortality Report*. Boston: Department of Developmental Services, Executive Office of Health and Human Services, Commonwealth of Massachusetts.

Lauer, E. (2012). *2009 Mortality Report*. Boston: Department of Developmental Services, Executive Office of Health and Human Services, Commonwealth of Massachusetts.

Lavis, D., Cullen, P. and Roy, A. (1997). Identification of hearing impairment in people with a learning disability: From questioning to testing. *British Journal of Learning Disabilities*, 25, 100–5.

Law, C. (2010). Policy and evidence-based public health. In A. Killoran and M. P. Kelly (eds.), *Evidence-based Public Health: Effectiveness and Efficiency*. Oxford University Press, pp. 27–39.

Lawn, S. and Pols, R. (2005). Smoking bans in psychiatric inpatient settings? A review of the research. *Australian and New Zealand Journal of Psychiatry*, 39, 866–85.

Lennox, N., Bain, C., Rey-Conde, T. et al. (2007). Effects of a comprehensive health assessment programme for Australian adults with intellectual disability: A cluster randomized trial. *International Journal of Epidemiology*, 36, 139–46. DOI: 10.1093/ije/dyl254.

Lennox, N., Bain, C., Rey-Conde, T. et al. (2010). Cluster randomized-controlled trial of interventions to improve health for adults with intellectual disability who live in private dwellings. *Journal of Applied Research in Intellectual Disabilities*, 23, 303–11.

Lennox, N., Terrace, R., Ware, R. et al. (2011). Effects of health screening for adults with intellectual disability: A pooled analysis. *British Journal of General Practice*, 61, 193–6.

Leonard, H., Nassar, N., Bourke, J. et al. (2008). Relation between intrauterine growth and subsequent intellectual disability in a ten-year population cohort of children in Western Australia. *American Journal of Epidemiology*, 167, 103–11.

Leonard, H., Petterson, B., Bower, C. and Sanders, R. (2003). Prevalence of intellectual disability in Western Australia. *Paediatric and Perinatal Epidemiology*, 17, 58–67.

Leonard, H., Petterson, B., De Klerk, N. et al. (2005). Association of sociodemographic characteristics of children with intellectual disability in Western Australia. *Social Science and Medicine*, 60, 1499–513.

Leonard, H. and Wen, X. (2002). The epidemiology of mental retardation: Challenges and opportunities in the new millennium. *Mental Retardation and Developmental Disabilities Research Reviews*, 8, 117–34.

Leventhal, T. and Newman, S. (2010). Housing and child development. *Children and Youth Services Review*, 32, 1165–74.

Lhatoo, S. D., Johnson, A. L., Goodridge, D. M. et al. (2001). Mortality in epilepsy in the first 11 to 14 years after diagnosis: Multivariate analysis of a long-term, prospective, population-based cohort. *Annals of Neurology*, 49(3), 336–44.

Lin, E., Balogh, R., Cobigo, V. et al. (2013). Using administrative health data to identify individuals with intellectual and developmental disabilities: A comparison of algorithms. *Journal of Intellectual Disabilities Research*, 57(5), 462–77.

Lin, J.-D., Lin, P.-Y., Lin, L.-P. (2010a). Universal hepatitis B vaccination coverage in children and adolescents with intellectual disabilities. *Research in Developmental Disabilities*, 31, 7.

Lin, L.-P., Lin, J.-D., Sung, C.-L., Liu, T.-W., Liu, Y.-L., Chen, L.-M., Chu, C.M. (2010b). Papanicolaou smear screening of women with intellectual disabilities: A cross-sectional survey in Taiwan. *Research in Developmental Disabilities*, 31, 7.

Linehan, C., Walsh, P. N., van Schrojenstein Lantman-deValk, H. et al. (2009). Are people with intellectual disabilities represented in European public health surveys? *Journal of Applied Research in Intellectual Disabilities*, 22, 409–20.

Livingston, J. D. and Boyd, J. E. (2010). Correlates and consequences of internalized stigma for people living with mental illness: A systematic review and meta-analysis. *Scal Science and Medicine*, 71, 2150–61.

Llewellyn, G., Emerson, E., Madden, R. and Honey, A. (2012). *The Well-Being of Children with Disabilities in the Asia Pacific Region: An Analysis of UNICEF MICS 3 Survey Data from Bangladesh, Laos PDR, Mongolia and Thailand*. Sydney: Centre for Disability Research and Policy, University of Sydney.

Llewellyn, G., McConnell, D., Gething, L., Cant, R. and Kendig, H. (2010). Health status and coping strategies among older parent-carers of adults with intellectual disabilities in an Australian sample. *Research in Developmental Disabilities*, 31, 1176–86.

Lloyd, M., Temple, V. A. and Foley, J. T. (2012). International BMI comparison of children and youth with intellectual disabilities participating in Special Olympics. *Research in Developmental Disabilities*, 33, 1708–14.

London Health Observatory. (Undated) www.lho.org.uk/LHO_Topics/Data/Methodology_and_Sources/AgeStandardisedRates.aspx.

Lorenc, T., Petticrew, M., Welch, V. and Tugwell, P. (2013). What types of interventions generate inequalities? Evidence from systematic reviews. *Journal of Epidemiology and Community Health*, 67, 190–3.

Louhiala, P. (2004). *Preventing Intellectual Disability: Ethical and Clinical Issues*. Cambridge University Press.

Lowe, K., Allen, D., Jones, E. et al. (2007). Challenging behaviours: Prevalence and topographies. *Journal of Intellectual Disability Research*, 51(8), 625–36.

Ludbrook, A. (2010). Fiscal policy and health-related behaviours. In A. Killoran and M. P. Kelly (eds.), *Evidence-based Public Health: Effectiveness and Efficiency*. Oxford: University Press, pp. 313–24.

Lund, C., Breen, A., Flisher, A. J. et al. (2010). Poverty and common mental disorders in low- and middle-income countries: A systematic review. *Social Science and Medicine*, 71, 517–28.

Lundeby, H. and Tøssebro, J. (2008). Family structure in Norwegian families with children with disabilities. *Journal of Applied Research in Intellectual Disabilities*, 21, 246–56.

Lunsky, Y., Lin, E., Balogh, R. et al. (2012). Emergency department visits and use of outpatient physican services by adults with developmental disability and psychiatric disorder. *Canadian Journal of Psychiatry*, 57, 601–7.

Luthar, S. S. (ed.). (2003). *Resilience and Vulnerability: Adaptation in the Context of Childhood Adversities*. Cambridge University Press.

Luthar, S. S. (2006). Resilience in development: A synthesis of research across five decades. In D. Cicchetti and D. J. Cohen (eds.), *Developmental Psychopathology, Vol. 3: Risk, Disorder, and Adaptation*. Hoboken, NJ: John Wiley and Sons, pp. 739–95.

Luthar, S. S. and Brown, P. J. (2007). Maximizing resilience through diverse levels of inquiry: Prevailing paradigms, possibilities, and priorities for the future. *Development and Psychopathology*, 19, 931–55.

Luthar, S. S., Sawyer, J. and Brown, P. (2006). Conceptual issues in studies of resilience. Past, present, and future research. *Annals of the New York Academy of Sciences*, 1094, 105–15.

Luttikhuis, H. O. B., Baur, L., Jansen, H. et al. (2009). Interventions for treating obesity in children. *Cochrane Database of Systematic Reviews*, CD001872.

MacDonald, E. E. and Hastings, R. P. (2010). Fathers of children with developmental disabilities. In M. E. Lamb (ed.), *The Role of the Father in Child Development*, 5th edn. Chichester: Wiley, pp. 486–516.

Mackenbach, J. and Bakker, M. (2002). *Reducing Inequalities in Health: A European Perspective*. London and New York: Routledge.

Mackenbach, J. P. (2012). The persistence of health inequalities in modern welfare states: The explanation of a paradox. *Social Science and Medicine*, 75, 761–9.

Madden, R., Ferreira, M., Einfeld, S. et al. (2012). New directions in healthcare and disability: The need for a shared understanding of human functioning. *Australian and New Zealand Journal of Public Health*. 36, 458–6.1 DOI: 10.1111/j.1753-6405.2012.00889.x.

Magana, S., Parish, S. L., Rose, R. A., Timberlake, M. and Swaine, J. G. (2012). Racial and ethnic disparities in quality of healthcare among children with autism and other developmental disabilities. *Intellectual and Developmental Disabilities*, 50, 287–99.

Mani, C. (1988). Hypothyroidism in Down's syndrome. *British Journal of Psychiatry*, 153, 102–4.

March, P. (1991). How do people with a mild/moderate mental handicap conceptualise physical illness and its cause? *British Journal of Mental Subnormality*, 37, 80–91.

Margalit, M. (2004). Loneliness and developmental disabilities: Cognitive and affective processing abilities. *International Review of Research in Mental Retardation*, 28, 225–53.

Marks, B. S., Sisirak, J., Heller, T. and Wagner, M. (2010). Evaluation of community-based health promotion programs for Special Olympics athletes. *Journal of Policy and Practice in Intellectual Disabilities*, 7, 119–29.

Marmot, M. (2005). Social determinants of health inequalities. *Lancet*, 365, 1099–104.

Marmot, M. and on behalf of the Commission on Social Determinants of Health. (2007). Achieving health equity: From root causes to fair outcomes. *Lancet*, 370, 1153–63.

Marmot, M., Smith, G., Stansfeld, S. et al. (1991). Health inequalities among British civil servants: The Whitehall II study. *Lancet*, 337, 1387–93.

Marmot, M. and Wilkinson, R. G. (eds.). (2006). *Social Determinants of Health* (2nd edn). Oxford University Press.

Martin, E., McKenzie, K., Newman, E., Bowden, K. and Morris, P. G. (2011). Care staff intentions to support adults with an intellectual disability to engage in physical activity: An application of the Theory of Planned Behaviour. *Research in Developmental Disabilities*, 32, 2535–41.

Masten, A. S. (2001). Ordinary magic: Resilience processes in development. *American Psychologist*, 56, 227–38.

Matthews, K. A., Gallo, L. C. and Taylor, S. E. (2010). Are psychosocial factors mediators of socio-economic status and health connections? A progress report and blueprint for the future. *Annals of the New York Academy of Sciences*, 1186, 146–73.

Matthews, T., Weston, N., Baxter, H., Felce, D. and Kerr, M. (2008). A general practice-based prevalence study of epilepsy among adults with intellectual disabilities and of its association with psychiatric disorder, behaviour disturbance and carer stress. *Journal of Intellectual Disability Research*, 52(2), 163–73.

Maughan, B., Collishaw, S. and Pickles, A. (1999). Mild mental retardation: Psychosocial functioning in adulthood. *Psychological Medicine*, 29, 351–66.

Maulik, P. K., Mascarenhas, M. N., Mathers, C. D., Dua, T. and Saxena, S. (2011). Prevalence of intellectual disability: A meta-analysis of population-based studies. *Research in Developmental Disabilities*, 32, 419–36.

Mayet, S., Farrell, M., Ferri, M., Amato, L., Davoli, M. Psychosocial treatment for opiate abuse and dependence. *Cochrane Database of Systematic Reviews*, 2005, Issue 1. Art. No.: CD004330. DOI: 10.1002/14651858.CD004330.pub2. Online: http://summaries. cochrane.org/CD004330/currently-there-is-not-enough-evidence-to-conclude-that-psychosocial-treatments-alone-are-adequate-to-treat-people-with-opiate-abuse-and-dependence.#sthash.xex0eOCz.dpuf

Mays, V. M., Cochran, S. D. and Barnes, N. W. (2007). Race, race-based discrimination, and health outcomes among African Americans. *Annual Review of Psychology*, 58, 201–25.

McCarthy, J., Hemmings, C., Kravariti, E. et al. (2010). Challenging behavior and co-morbid psychopathology in adults with intellectual disability and autism spectrum disorders. *Research in Developmental Disabilities*, 31, 362–6.

McConnell, D., Llewellyn, G., Mayes, R., Russo, D. and Honey, A. (2003). Developmental profiles of children born to mothers with intellectual disability. *Journal of Intellectual and Developmental Disability*, 28, 122–34.

McConnell, D., Mayes, R. and Llewellyn, G. (2008). Women with intellectual disability at risk of adverse pregnancy and birth outcomes. *Journal of Intellectual Disability Research*, 52, 529–35.

McDermott, S. W., Whitner, W., Thomas-Koger, M. et al. (2012). An efficacy trial of 'Steps to Your Health', a health promotion programme for adults with intellectual disability. *Health Education Journal*, 71(3), 278–90.

McDowell, I. (2006). *Measuring Health, 3rd edn.* Oxford University Press.

McEwen, B. S. and Gianaros, P. J. (2010). Central role of the brain in stress and adaptation: Links to socio-economic status, health, and disease. *Annals of the New York Academy of Sciences*, 1186, 190–222.

McGillicuddy, N. (2006a). A review of substance use research among those with mental retardation. *Mental Retardation and Developmental Disabilities Research Reviews*, 12, 7.

McGillicuddy, N. (2006b). A review of substance use research among those with mental retardation. *Mental Retardation and Developmental Disability Research Reviews*, 12, 41–7.

McGillicuddy, N. B. and Blane, H. (1999). Substance use in individuals with mental retardation. *Addictive Behaviors*, 24(6), 869–78.

McGlade, A., Bickerstaff, D., Lindsay, J., McConkey, R. and Jackson, J. (2010). Making a difference. Visual health needs of people with a learning disability. *British Journal of Learning Disabilities*, 38, 187–93.

McGuigan, S. M., Hollins, S. and Attard, M. (1995). Age-specific standardised mortality rates in people with learning disability. *Journal of Intellectual Disability Research*, 39, 527–31.

McGuire, B. E., Daly, P. and Smyth, F. (2010). Chronic pain in people with an intellectual disability: Under-recognised and under-treated? *Journal of Intellectual Disability Research*, 54, 240–5.

McInnis, E. E., Hills, A. and Chapman, M. J. (2011). Eligibility for statutory learning disability services in the north-west of England. Right or luxury? Findings from a pilot study. *British Journal of Learning Disabilities*, 40, 177–86.

McQueen, P. C., Spence, M. W., Garner, J. B., Pereira, L. H. and Winsor, E. J. T. (1987). Prevalence of major mental retardation and associated disabilities in the Canadian Maritime provinces. *American Journal on Mental Deficiency*, 91, 460–6.

Megret, F. (2008). The disabilities convention: Human rights of persons with disabilities or disability rights? *Human Rights Quarterly*, 30, 494–516.

Melhuish, E., Belsky, J. and Barnes, J. (2010). Child health and well-being in the early years: The National Evaluation of Sure Start. In A. Killoran and A. P. Kelly (eds.), *Evidence-based Public Health: Effectiveness and Efficiency*. Oxford University Press, pp. 203–14.

Melville, C., Hamilton, S., Hankey, C., Miller, S. and Boyle, S. (2007). The prevalence and determinants of obesity in adults with intellectual disabilities. *Obesity Reviews*, 8, 223–30.

Melville, C., Hamilton, S., Miller, S. et al. (2009). Carer knowledge and perceptions of healthy lifestyles for adults with intellectual disabilities. *Journal of Applied Research in Intellectual Disabilities*, 22, 298–306.

Melville, C. A., Cooper, S. A., McGrother, C. W., Thorp, C. F. and Collacott, R. (2005). Obesity in adults with Down syndrome: A case-control study. *Journal of Intellectual Disability Research*, 49, 125–33.

Melville, C. A., Cooper, S. A., Morrison, J. et al. (2008). The prevalence and determinants of obesity in adults with intellectual disabilities. *Journal of Applied Research in Intellectual Disabilities*, 21, 425–37.

Mencap. (2007). *Death by Indifference*. London: Mencap.

Mencap. (2012a). *Death by Indifference: 74 deaths and Counting. A Progress Report 5 Years On*. London: Mencap.

Mencap. (2012b). *Out of Sight: Stopping the Neglect and Abuse of People with a Learning Disability*. London: Mencap.

Mencap and Challenging Behaviour Foundation. (2012). *Out of Sight: Stopping the Neglect and Abuse of People with a Learning Disability*. London: Mencap and Challenging Behaviour Foundation.

Mergler, S., Evenhuis, H. M., Boot, A. M. et al. (2009). Epidemiology of low bone mineral density and fractures in children with severe cerebral palsy: A systematic review. *Developmental Medicine and Child Neurology*, 51, 773–8.

Merrick, J. and Morad, M. (2010). Cardiovascular disease. In J. O'Hara, J. E. McCarthy and N. Bouras (eds.), *Intellectual Disability and Ill Health: A Review of the Evidence*. Cambridge University Press, pp. 73–7.

Messent, P. R., Cooke, C. B. and Long, J. (1998). Physical activity, exercise and health of adults with mild and moderate learning disabilities. *British Journal of Learning Disabilities*, 26, 17–22.

Meyers, D. G., Neuberger, J. S. and He, J. (2009). Cardiovascular effect of bans on smoking in public places. *Journal of the American College of Cardiology*, 54, 1249–55.

Michael, J. (2008). *Healthcare for All: Report of the Independent Inquiry into Access to Healthcare for People with Learning Disabilities*. London: Independent Inquiry into Access to Healthcare for People with Learning Disabilities.

Miller, G., Chen, E. and Parker, K. (2011). Psychological stress in childhood and susceptibility to the chronic diseases of aging: Moving toward a model of behavioral and biological mechanisms. *Psychological Bulletin*, 137, 959–97.

Mir, G., Nocon, A., Ahmad, W. and Jones, L. (2004). *Learning Difficulties and Ethnicity*. London: Department of Health.

Mohaupt, S. (2009). Resilience and social exclusion. *Social Policy and Society*, 8, 63–71.

Molyneux, P., Emerson, E. and Caine, A. (1999). Prescription of psychotropic medication to people with intellectual disabilities in primary healthcare settings. *Journal of Applied Research in Intellectual Disabilities*, 12, 46–57.

Mont, D. (2007). *Measuring Disability Prevalence*. Washington, DC: The World Bank.

Morgan, C. L., Ahmed, Z. and Kerr, M. P. (2000). Healthcare provision for people with a learning disability: Record-linkage study of epidemiology and factors contributing to hospital care uptake. *British Journal of Psychiatry*, 176, 37–41.

Morgan, C. L. and Kerr, M. P. (2002). Epilepsy and mortality: A record linkage study in a UK population. *Epilepsia*, 43(10), 1251–5.

Morgan, J. P., Minihan, P. M., Stark, P. C. et al. (2012). The oral health status of 4,732 adults with intellectual and developmental disabilities. *Journal of the American Dental Association*, 143, 838–46.

Morin, D., Merineau-Cote, J., Ouellette-Kuntz, H., Tasse, M. J. and Kerr, M. (2012). A comparison of the prevalence of chronic disease among people with and without intellectual disability. *American Journal on Intellectual and Developmental Disabilities*, 117, 455–63.

Morin, D., Rivard, M., Crocker, A. G., Boursier, C. P. and Caron, J. (2013). Public attitudes towards intellectual disability: A multidimensional perspective. *Journal of Intellectual Disabilities Research*, 57, 279–92.

Murayama, H., Fujiwara, Y. and Kawachi, I. (2012). Social capital and health: A review of prospective multilevel studies. *Journal of Epidemiology*, 22, 179–87

Murphy, G. H., O'Callaghan, A. C. and Clare, I. C. H. (2007). The impact of alleged abuse on behaviour in adults with severe intellectual disabilities. *Journal of Intellectual Disability Research*, 51, 741–9.

Murray, C. J. L. and Lopez, A. D. (eds.). (1996). *The Global Burden of Disease: A Comprehensive Assessment of Mortality and Disability from Diseases, Injuries, and Risk Factors in 1990 and Projected to 2020*. Cambridge, MA: Harvard University Press.

Murray, S. and Powell, A. (2008). *Sexual Assault and Adults with a Disability: Enabling Recognition, Disclosure and a Just Response* (ACSSA Issues Paper No. 9). Melbourne: Australian Institute of Family Studies.

Nashef, L., Fish, D. R., Garner, S., Sander, J. W. and Shorvon, S. D. (1995). Sudden death in epilepsy: A study of incidence in a young cohort with epilepsy and learning difficulty. *Epilepsia*, 36(12), 1187–94.

National Center on Birth Defects and Developmental Disabilities. (2010). *U.S. Surveillance of Health of People with Intellectual Disabilities: A White Paper*. Atlanta: Centers for Disease Control and Prevention.

National Equality Panel. (2010). *An Anatomy of Economic Inequality in the UK*. London: Government Equalities Office.

Neligan, A., Bell, G. S., Johnson, A. L. et al. (2011). The long-term risk of premature mortality in people with epilepsy. *Brain*, 134(2), 388–95. DOI: 10.1093/brain/awq378.

Newschaffer, C. J., Croen, L. A., Daniels, J. et al. (2007). The epidemiology of autism spectrum disorders. *Annual Review of Public Health*, 28, 235–58.

NHS Health Scotland. (2004). *People with Learning Disabilities in Scotland: Health Needs Assessment Report*. Glasgow: NHS Health Scotland.

NHS Information Centre for Health and Social Care. (2012a). *Community Care Statistics 2010–11: Social Services Activity Report, England*. Leeds: NHS Information Centre for Health and Social Care.

NHS Information Centre for Health and Social Care. (2012b). *Personal Social Services: Expenditure and Unit Costs – England 2010-11 – Final Release.* Leeds: NHS Information Centre for Health and Social Care.

Nielsen, L. S., Skov, L. and Jensen, H. (2007a). Visual dysfunctions and ocular disorders in children with developmental delay. I Prevalence, diagnoses and aetiology of visual impairment. *Acta Ophthalmologica Scandinavica*, 85, 149–56.

Nielsen, L. S., Skov, L. and Jensen, H. (2007b). Visual dysfunctions and ocular disorders in children with developmental delay. II Aspects of refractive errors, strabismus and contrast sensitivity. *Acta Ophthalmologica Scandinavica*, 85, 419–26.

Noble, S. E., Leyland, K., Findlay, C. A. et al. (2000). School-based screening for hypothyroidism in Down's syndrome by dried blood spot TSH measurement. *Archive of Diseases of Childhood*, 82, 27–31.

Nocon, A. (2006). *Equal Treatment – Closing the Gap: Background Evidence for the DRC's Formal Investigation into Health Inequalities Experienced by People with Learning Disabilities or Mental Health Problems.* Manchester: Disability Rights Commission.

Norwood, K. W. and Slayton, R. L. (2013). Oral healthcare for children with developmental disabilities. *Pediatrics*, 131, 614–19.

Nussbaum, M. (2009). The capabilities of people with cognitive disabilities. *Metaphilosophy*, 40(3–4), 331–51.

Nussbaum, M. C. (2011). *Creating Capabilities: The Human Development Approach.* Cambridge, MA: Belknap Press of Harvard University Press.

O'Hara, J. (2010). Healthcare and intellectual disability. In J. O'Hara, J. E. McCarthy and N. Bouras (eds.), *Intellectual Disability and Ill Health: A Review of the Evidence.* Cambridge University Press, pp. 3–16.

O'Hara, J., McCarthy, J. and Bouras, N. (eds.). (2010a). *Intellectual Disability and Ill Health.* Cambridge University Press.

O'Hara, J., McCarthy, J. E. and Bouras, N. (2010b). *Intellectual Disability and Ill Health: A Review of the Evidence.* Cambridge University Press.

Oberlander, T. F., Burkitt, C. C., Symons, F. J. and Johnston, C. (2012). Sensory functions: Pain (B280–B289). In A. Majnemer (ed.), *Measures for Children with Developmental Disabilities.* Plymouth: MacKeith Press, pp. 170–80.

Obi, O., Braun, K. V., Baio, J., Drews-Botsch, C., Devine, O., & Yeargin-Allsopp, M. (2011). Effect of incorporating adaptive functioning scores on the prevalence of intellectual disability. *American Journal on Intellectual and Developmental Disabilities,* 116(5), 360–370.

ODI. (2011). *Disability Prevalence Estimates 2010/11.* London: Department for Work and Pensions.

Oeseburg, B., Dijkstra, G. J., Groothoff, J. W. et al. (2011). Prevalence of chronic health conditions in children with intellectual disability: A systematic literature review. *Intellectual and Developmental Disabilities*, 49, 59–85.

Office for National Statistics. (2011). *National Population Projections 2010-based Statistical Bulletin.* London: Office for National Statistics.

Office for National Statistics. (2012). *Deaths Registered in England and Wales (Series DR), 2011.* Swansea: Office for National Statistics.

Officer, A. and Groce, N. E. (2009). Key concepts in disability. *Lancet*, 374, 1795–6.

Oliver, C. and Richards, C. (2010). Self-injurious behaviour in people with intellectual disability. *Current Opinion in Psychiatry*, 23, 412–16.

Open Society Institute. (2006). *Access to Education and Employment for People with Intellectual Disabilities: Overview of the Situation in Central and Eastern Europe*. Budapest: Open Society Mental Health Initiative.

Organisation for Economic Co-operation and Development. (2013). *OECD Guidelines on Measuring Subjective Well-being*. Paris: Organisation for Economic Co-operation and Development.

Osborn, D. P. J., Horsfall, L., Hassiotis, A. et al. (2012). Access to cancer screening in people with learning disabilities in the UK: Cohort study in the Health Improvement Network, a primary care research database. *PLoS ONE*, 7. DOI: 10.1371/journal.pone.0043841.

Ouellette-Kuntz, H. (2005). Understanding health disparities and inequities faced by individuals with intellectual disabilities. *Journal of Applied Research in Intellectual Disabilities*, 18, 113–21.

Owen, D. M., Hastings, R. P., Noone, S. J. et al. (2004). Life events as correlates of problem behavior and mental health in a residential population of adults with developmental disabilities. *Research in Developmental Disabilities*, 25, 309–20.

Owens, J., Dyer, T. A. and Mistry, K. (2010). People with learning disabilities and specialist services. *British Dental Journal*, 208, 203–5.

Paasche-Orlow, M. K., Parker, R. M., Gazmararian, J. A., Nielsen-Bohlman, L. T. and Rudd, R. R. (2005). The prevalence of limited health literacy. *Journal of General Internal Medicine*, 20, 175–84.

Paradies, Y. (2006). A systematic review of empirical research on self-reported racism and health. *International Journal of Epidemiology*, 35, 888–901.

Parish, S. L. and Cloud, J. M. (2006). Financial well-being of young children with disabilities and their families. *Social Work*, 51(3), 223–32.

Parish, S. L., Rose, R. A., Andrews, M. E., Grinstein-Weiss, M. and Richman, E. L. (2008). Material hardship in US families raising children with disabilities. *Exceptional Children*, 75(1), 71–92.

Parish, S. L., Swaine, J. G., Luken, K., Rose, R. A. and Dababnah, S. (2012). Cervical and breast cancer-screening knowledge of women with developmental disabilities. *Intellectual and Developmental Disabilities*, 50, 79–91.

Patja, K., Iivanainen, M., Vesala, H., Oksansn, H. and Ruoppila, I. (2000). Life expectancy of people with intellectual disability: A 35-year follow-up study. *Journal of Intellectual Disability Research*, 44, 591–9.

Patja, K., Mölsä, P. and Iivanainen, M. (2001). Cause-specific mortality of people with intellectual disability in a population-based, 35-year follow-up study. *Journal of Intellectual Disability Research*, 45(1), 30–40.

Pearson, V., Davis, C., Ruoff, C. and Dyer, J. (1998). Only one quarter of women with learning disability in Exeter have cervical screening. *British Medical Journal*, 316, 1979.

Peine, H. A. D., Darvish, R., Blacklock, H., Osborne, J. G. and Jensen, W. R. (1998). Non-aversive reduction of cigarette smoking in two adult men in a residential setting. *Journal of Behavior Therapy*, 29, 55–65.

Perry, D., Hammond, L., Marston, G., Gaskell, S. and Eva, J. (2011). *Caring for the Physical and Mental Health of People with Learning Disabilities*. London: Jessica Kingsley.

Perry, J. (2004). Interviewing people with intellectual disabilities. In E. Emerson, C. Hatton, T. Thompson and T. Parmenter (eds.), *The International Handbook of Applied Research in Intellectual Disabilities*. Chichester: Wiley.

Peate, I. and Maloret, P. (2007). Testicular self-examination: the person with learning disabilities. *British Journal of Nursing,* 16, 5.

Petrone, L. R. (2012). Osteoporosis in adults with intellectual disabilities. *Southern Medical Journal,* 105, 87–92.

Piachaud, J. and Rohde, J. (1998). Screening for breast cancer is necessary in patients with learning disability. *British Medical Journal,* 316, 1979.

Piachaud, J., Rohde, J. and Pasupathy, A. (1998). Health screening for people with Down's syndrome. *Journal of Intellectual Disability Research,* 42, 341–5.

Pickett, K. E. and Wilkinson, R. G. (2007). Child well-being and income inequality in rich societies: Ecological cross-sectional study. *British Medical Journal,* 335, 1080–6.

Pinborough-Zimmerman, J., Satterfield, R., Miller, J. et al. (2007). Communication disorders: Prevalence and comorbid intellectual disability, autism, and emotional/behavioral disorders. *American Journal of Speech-Language Pathology,* 16, 359–67.

Popham, F., Dibben, C. and Bambra, C. (2013). Are health inequalities really not the smallest in the Nordic welfare states? A comparison of mortality inequality in 37 countries. *Journal of Epidemiology and Community Health,* 67, 412–18.

Pound, E. C., Coleman, T., Adams, C., Ferguson, J. and Bauld, L. (2005). Targeting smokers from disadvantaged groups: The influence of targets and policy statements. *Addiction,* 100(Suppl. 2), 28–35.

Power, M. J., Green, A. M. and Grp, W. H.-D. (2010). Development of the WHOQOL disabilities module. *Quality of Life Research,* 19(4), 571–84. DOI: 10.1007/s11136-010-9616-6.

Pownall, J. D., Jahoda, A., Hastings, R. P. (2012). Sexuality and sex education of adolescents with intellectual disability: Mothers' attitudes, experiences, and support needs. *Intellectual and Developmental Disabilities,* 50(2), 15.

Prasher, V. and Janicki, M. P. (eds.). (2003). *Physical Health of Adults with Intellectual Disabilities.* Oxford: Blackwell.

Prasher, V., Ninan, S. and Haque, S. (2011). Fifteen-year follow-up of thyroid status in adults with Down syndrome. *Journal of Intellectual Disability Research,* 55, 392–6.

Prasher, V. P. (1995). Overweight and obesity amongst Down's syndrome adults. *Journal of Intellectual Disability Research,* 39, 437–41.

Prosser, H. and Bromley, J. (2012). Interviewing people with intellectual disability, 2nd edn. In E. Emerson, C. Hatton, K. Dickson, R. Gone, A. Caine and J. Bromley (eds.), *Clinical Psychology and People with Intellectual Disabilities.* Chichester: Wiley, pp. 107–20.

Proto, C., Romualdi, D., Cento, R. M. et al. (2007). Free and total leptin serum levels and soluble leptin receptor levels in two models of genetic obesity: The Prader-Willi and the Down syndromes. *Metabolism: Clinical and Experimental,* 56, 1076–80.

Prout, H. T. B. (2011). The effectiveness of psychotherapy for persons with intellectual disabilities. In R. J. Fletcher (ed.), *Psychotherapy for Individuals with Intellectual Disability.* Kingston, NY: National Association of Developmental Disabilities Press, pp. 265–87.

Prout, R. and Nowak-Drabik, K.M. (2003). Psychotherapy with persons who have mental retardation: An evaluation of effectiveness. *American Journal on Mental Retardation,* 108, 14.

Pueschel, S. M., Jackson, I. M. D. and Giesswein, P. (1991). Thyroid function in Down's Syndrome. *Research in Developmental Disabilities,* 12, 287–96.

Purcell, M., Morris, I. and McConkey, R. (1999). Staff perceptions of the communicative competence of adult persons with intellectual disabilities. *British Journal of Developmental Disabilities*, 45, 16–25.

Puri, B. K., Lekh, S. K., Langa, A., Zaman, R. and Singh, I. (1995). Mortality in a hospitalized mentally handicapped population: A 10-year survey. *Journal of Intellectual Disability Research*, 39, 442–6.

Radhakrishnan, V. (2010). Otorhinolaryngologal disorders. In J. O'Hara, J. E. McCarthy and N. Bouras (eds.), *Intellectual Disability and Ill Health: A Review of the Evidence*. Cambridge University Press, pp. 137–45.

Rani, F. A., Byrne, P., Cranswick, N., Murray, M. L. and Wong, I. C. K. (2010). Mortality in children and adolescents prescribed antipsychotic medication: A retrospective cohort study using the UK General Practice Research Database. *Drug Safety*, 34(9), 773–81.

Rantakallio, P. and von Wendt, L. (1986). Mental retardation and subnormality in a birth cohort of 12,000 children in Northern Finland. *American Journal of Mental Deficiency*, 90, 380–7.

Rasmussen, S. A., Wong, L. Y., Correa, A., Gambrell, D. and Friedman, J. M. (2006). Survival in infants with Down syndrome, Metropolitan Atlanta, 1979–1998. *Journal of Pediatrics*, 148, 806–12.

Ravesloot, C. R., Ruggiero, C., Ipsen, C. et al. (2011). Disability and health behavior change. *Disability and Health Journal*, 4, 19–23.

Read, J., Blackburn, C. and Spencer, N. (2012). Disabled children and their families: A decade of policy change. *Children and Society*, 26, 223–333.

Rechel, B., Kennedy, C., McKee, M. and Rechel, B. (2011). The Soviet legacy in diagnosis and treatment: Implications for population health. *Journal of Public Health Policy*, 32, 293–304.

Reichard, A. and Stolzle, H. (2011). Diabetes among adults with cognitive limitations compared to individuals with no cognitive disabilities. *Intellectual and Developmental Disabilities*, 49, 141–54.

Reid, K. A., Smiley, E. and Cooper, S. A. (2011). Prevalence and associations of anxiety disorders in adults with intellectual disabilities. *Journal of Intellectual Disability Research*, 55, 172–81.

Renz, A., Ide, M., Newton, T., Robinson, P., Smith, D. (2007). Psychological interventions to improve adherence to oral hygiene instructions in adults with periodontal disease. *Cochrane Database of Systematic Reviews* 2007, Issue 2. Art. No.: CD005097. DOI: 10.1002/14651858.CD005097.pub2.

Reynolds, F., Stanistreet, D. and Elton, P. (2008). Women with learning disabilities and access to cervical screening: Retrospective cohort study using case control methods. *BMC Public Health*, 8, 30.

Richards, D. A.; Borglin, G. (2011). Implementation of psychological therapies for anxiety and depression in routine practice: Two year prospective cohort study. *Journal of Affective Disorders*, 10.

Rimmer, J. H., Braddock, D. and Marks, B. (1995). Health characteristics and behaviors of adults with mental retardation residing in three living arrangements. *Research in Developmental Disabilities*, 16, 489–99.

Rippon, L. (2010). Inpatient services for children and young people with an intellectual disability. *Advances in Mental Health and Intellectual Disabilities*, 4, 4–8.

Roberts, H., Copeland, A., Glover, G., Hatton, C. and Baines, S. (2012). *Learning Disability Partnership Board Progress Reports 2010/11: A Thematic Analysis*. Durham: Learning Disabilities Public Health Observatory.

Robertson, J., Emerson, E., Gregory, N. et al. (2000a). Receipt of psychotropic medication by people with intellectual disability in residential settings. *Journal of Intellectual Disability Research*, 44, 666–76.

Robertson, J., Emerson, E., Gregory, N. et al. (2000b). Lifestyle-related risk factors for poor health in residential settings for people with intellectual disabilities. *Research in Developmental Disabilities*, 21, 469–86.

Robertson, J., Emerson, E., Gregory, N. et al. (2001). Social networks of people with mental retardation in residential settings. *Mental Retardation*, 39, 201–14.

Robertson, J., Emerson, E., Pinkney, L. et al. (2005). Treatment and management of challenging behaviour in congregate and noncongregate community-based supported accommodation. *Journal of Intellectual Disability Research*, 49, 63–72.

Robertson, J., Roberts, H. and Emerson, E. (2010). *Health Checks for People with Learning Disabilities: Systematic Review of Impact*. Durham: Improving Health and Lives: Learning Disability Observatory.

Robertson, J., Roberts, H., Emerson, E., Turner, S. and Greig, R. (2011). The impact of health checks for people with intellectual disabilities: A systematic review of evidence. *Journal of Intellectual Disabilities Research*, 55, 1009–19.

Rodgers, J. (1998). 'Whatever's on her plate': food in the lives of people with learning disabilities. *British Journal of Learning Disabilities*, 26, 13–16.

Rodgers, J., Lipscombe, J. and Santer, M. (2006). Menstrual problems experienced by women with learning disabilities. *Journal of Applied Research in Intellectual Disabilities*, 19, 364–73.

Roeleveld, N., Zielhuis, G. A. and Gabreels, F. (1997). The prevalence of mental retardation: A critical review of recent literature. *Developmental Medicine and Child Neurology*, 39, 125–32.

Rosen, J. W. and Burchard, S. N. (1990). Community activities and social support networks: A social comparison of adults with and adults without mental retardation. *Education and Training in Mental Retardation*, 25, 193–204.

Roulstone, A. and Mason-Bish, H. (eds.). (2012). *Disability, Hate Crime and Violence*. London: Routledge.

Roux, A. V. D. and Mair, C. (2010). Neighborhoods and health. *Annals of the New York Academy of Sciences*, 1186, 125–45.

Roy, A., Martin, D. M. and Wells, M. B. (1997). Health gain through screening – mental health: Developing primary healthcare services for people with an intellectual disability. *Journal of Intellectual and Developmental Disability*, 22, 227–39.

Royal College of Psychiatrists. (2001). *DC-LD: Diagnostic Criteria for Psychiatric Disorders for Use with Adults with Learning Disabilities/Mental Retardation (Occasional Paper OP 48)*. London: Gaskell.

Royal College of Psychiatrists, British Psychological Society and Royal College of Speech and Language Therapists. (2007). *Clinical and Service Guidelines for Supporting People with Learning Disabilities Who are at Risk of Receiving Abusive or Restrictive Practices*. London: Royal College of Psychiatrists.

Ruedrich, S. (2010). Mental illness. In J. O'Hara, J. E. McCarthy and N. Bouras (eds.), *Intellectual Disability and Ill Health: A Review of the Evidence*. Cambridge University Press, pp. 165–77.

Rutter, M. (1979). Protective factors in children's responses to stress and disadvantage. In M. W. Kent and J. E. Rolf (eds.), *Primary Prevention of Psychopathology. III. Social Competence in Children*. Hanover, NH: University Press of New England, pp. 49–74.

Rutter, M. (1985). Resilience in the face of adversity: Protective factors and resistence to psychiatric disorders. *British Journal of Psychiatry*, 147, 589–611.

Rutter, M., Beckett, C., Castle, J. et al. (2009). Effects of profound early institutional deprivation: An overview of findings from a UK longitudinal study of Romanian adoptees. In G. M. Wrobel and E. Neil (eds.), *International Advances in Adoption Research for Practice*. Chichester: Wiley-Blackwell, pp. 147–67.

Samele, C., Seymour, L., Morris, B. et al. (2006). *A Formal Investigation into Health Inequalities Experienced by People with Learning Difficulties and People with Mental Health Problems: Area Studies Report*. London: The Sainsbury Centre for Mental Health.

Sandberg, S. and Rutter, M. (2008). Acute life stresses. In M. Rutter, D. Bishop, D. Pine, S. Scott, J. Stevenson, E. Taylor and A. Thapar (eds.), *Rutter's Child and Adolescent Psychiatry*. Oxford: Blackwell, pp. 392–408.

Sanders, L. M., Federico, S., Klass, P., Abrams, M. A. and Dreyer, B. (2009). Literacy and child health: A systematic review. *Archives of Pediatric and Adolescent Medicine*, 163, 131–40.

Scambler, S. (2012). Disabling conditions and disability theory. In N. Watson, A. Roulstone and C. Thomas (eds.), *Routledge Handbook of Disability Studies*. London: Routledge, pp. 136–50.

Scheepers, M., Kerr, M., O'Hara, D. et al. (2005). Reducing health disparity in people with intellectual disabilities: A report from the Health Issues Special Interest Research Group of the International Association for the Scientific Study of Intellectual Disabilities. *Journal of Policy and Practice in Intellectual Disabilities*, 2, 249–55.

Schieve, L. A., Gonzalez, V., Boulet, S. L. et al. (2012). Concurrent medical conditions and healthcare use and needs among children with learning and behavioral developmental disabilities, National Health Interview Survey, 2006–2010. *Research in Developmental Disabilities*, 33, 467–76.

Schoon, I. (2006). *Risk and Resilience: Adaptations in Changing Times*. Cambridge University Press.

Schupf, N., Zigman, W., Kapell, D. et al. (1997). Early menopause in women with Down's syndrome. *Journal of Intellectual Disability Research*, 41, 264–7.

Seekins, T. D., Kimpton, T., Peterson, J. et al. (2010). *Community-based Health Promotion Interventions for People with Disabilities: Results of a Scoping Review of the Literature*. Portland, OR: Rehabilitation Research and Training Center on Health and Wellness for Adults with Long-Term Disabilities.

Seeman, T. E. (1996). Social ties and health: The benefits of social integration. *Annals of Epidemiology*, 6, 442–51.

Seltzer, M. M., Floyd, F., Greenberg, J. et al. (2005). Life course impacts of mild intellectual deficits. *American Journal on Mental Retardation*, 110(6), 451–68.

Sen, A. (2001). *Development as Freedom*. Oxford University Press.

Sequeira, H. and Hollins, S. (2003). Clinical effects of sexual abuse on people with learning disability: Critical literature review. *British Journal of Psychiatry*, 182, 13–19.

Servais, L. (2006). Sexual health care in persons with intellectual disabilities. *Mental Retardation and Developmental Disabilities Research Reviews*, 12, 9.

Shahtahmasebi, S., Emerson, E., Berridge, D. and Lancaster, G. (2011). Child disability and the dynamics of family poverty, hardship and financial strain: Evidence from the UK. *Journal of Social Policy*, 40, 653–73.

Shakespeare, T. (2006). *Disability Rights and Wrongs*. London: Routledge.

Shattuck, P. T., Orsmond, G. I., Wagner, M. and Cooper, B. P. (2011). Participation in social activities among adolescents with an autism spectrum disorder. *PLoS 1*, 6(11), e27176. DOI:10.1371/journal.pone.0027176.

Shephard-Jones, K., Prout, H. T. and Kleinert, H. (2005). Quality of life dimensions for adults with developmental disabilities: A comparative study. *Mental Retardation*, 43(4), 281–91.

Sherrard, J., Tonge, B. J. and Ozanne-Smith, J. (2002). Injury risk in young people with intellectual disability. *Journal of Intellectual Disability Research*, 46, 6–16.

Sherry, M. (2010). *Disability Hate Crimes: Does Anyone Really Hate Disabled People?* Burlington: Ashgate.

Shogren, K. A., Wehmeyer, M. L., Reese, R. M. and O'Hara, D. (2006). Promoting self-determination in health and medical care: A critical component of addressing health disparities in people with intellectual disabilities. *Journal of Policy and Practice in Intellectual Disabilities*, 3, 105–13.

Shonkoff, J. P. (2010). Building a new biodevelopmental framework to guide the future of early childhood policy. *Child Development*, 81, 357–67.

Shonkoff, J. P., Boyce, W. T. and McEwen, B. S. (2009). Neuroscience, molecular biology, and the childhood roots of health disparities: Building a new framework for health promotion and disease prevention. *JAMA*, 301, 2252–9.

Simpson, C. G., Swicegood, P. R., Gaus, M. D. (2006). Nutrition and fitness curriculum: Designing instructional interventions for children with developmental disabilities. *Teaching Exceptional Children*, 38(6), 4.

Singer, G. H. (2006). Meta-analysis of comparative studies of depression in mothers of children with and without developmental disabilities. *American Journal on Mental Retardation*, 111(3), 155–69.

Singh, N. N. L., Lancioni, G. E., Winton, A. S. W. et al. (2011). Effects of a mindfulness-based smoking cessation program for an adult with mild intellectual disability. *Research in Developmental Disabilities*, 32, 1180–5.

Singleton, N., Bumpstead, R., O'Brien, M., Lee, A. and Meltzer, H. (2001). *Psychiatric Morbidity among Adults Living in Private Households, 2000*. London: The Stationery Office.

Sipes, M., Matson, J. L., Belva, B. et al. (2011). The relationship among side effects associated with anti-epileptic medications in those with intellectual disability. *Research in Developmental Disabilities*, 32, 1646–51.

Slayter, E. (2008). Understanding and overcoming barriers to substance abuse treatment access for people with mental retardation. *Journal of Social Work and Disability Rehabilitation*, 7(2), 18.

Slayter, E. (2010a). Demographic and clinical characteristics of people with intellectual disabilities with and without substance abuse disorders in a Medicaid population. *Intellectual and Developmental Disabilities*, 48(6), 15.

Slayter, E. (2010b). Not immune: Access to substance abuse treatment among Medicaid-covered youth with mental retardation. *Journal of Disability Policy Studies*, 20(4), 10.

Slevin, E., Truesdale-Kennedy, M., McConkey, R., Livingstone, B. and Fleming, P. (In press). Obesity and overweight in intellectually and non-intellectually disabled children. *Journal of Intellectual Disabilities Research*.

Smulders, E., Enkelaar, L., Weerdesteyn, V., Geurts, C. H. and van Schrojenstein Lantman-deValk, H. (In press). Falls in older persons with intellectual disabilities: Fall rate, circumstances and consequences. *Journal of Intellectual Disabilities Research*.

Snell, M. and Luckasson, R. (2009). Characteristics and needs of people with intellectual disability who have higher IQs. *Intellectual and Developmental Disabilities*, 47, 220–33.

Snell, M. E., Brady, N., McLean, L. et al. (2010). Twenty years of communication intervention research with indivuiduals who have severe intellectual and developmental disabilities. *American Journal on Intellectual and Developmental Disability*, 115, 364–80.

Stafford, M., Nazroo, J., Popay, J. and Whitehead, M. (2008). Tackling inequalities in health: Evaluating the New Deal for Communities initiative. *Journal of Epidemiology and Community Health*, 62, 298–304.

Stainland, L. (2011). *Public Perceptions of Disabled People: Evidence from the British Social Attitudes Survey 2009*. Sheffield: Office for Disability Issues.

Stalker, K. (2012). Theorizing the position of people with learning difficulties within disability studies: Progress and pitfalls. In N. Watson, A. Roulstone and C. Thomas (eds.), *Routledge Handbook of Disability Studies*. London: Routledge, pp. 122–35.

Stallard, P., Williams, L., Lenton, S. and Velleman, R. (2001). Pain in cognitively impaired, non-communicating children *Archive of Diseases of Childhood*, 85, 460–2.

Stancliffe, R. (2000). Proxy respondents and quality of life. *Evaluation and Programme Planning*, 23, 89–93.

Stancliffe, R. J. (2007). Loneliness and living arrangements. *Intellectual and Developmental Disabilities*, 45, 380–90.

Stancliffe, R. J., Lakin, K. C., Larson, S. A. et al. (2012). Demographic characteristics, health conditions, and residential service use in adults with Down Syndrome in 25 U.S. states. *Intellectual and Developmental Disabilities*, 50, 92–108.

Stanish, H. I. T. and Temple, V.-A. (2012). Efficacy of a peer-guided exercise programme for adolescents with intellectual disability. *Journal of Applied Research in Intellectual Disabilities*, 25, 319–28.

Stansfeld, S. A. (2006). Social support and social cohesion. In M. Marmot and R. G. Wilkinson (eds.), *Social Determinants of Health*. Oxford University Press, pp. 148–71.

Stead, L. F. and Lancaster, L. T. (2009). Group behaviour therapy programmes for smoking cessation. *Cochrane Database of Systemic Reviews*, CD001007.

Stein, K. and Ball, D. (1999). Contact between people with learning disability and general practitioners: A cross-sectional case note survey. *Journal of Public Medicine*, 21, 192–8.

Steinberg, M. L., Heimlich, H. L. and Williams, J. M. (2009). Tobacco use among individuals with intellectual or developmental disabilities: A brief review. *Intellectual and Developmental Disabilities*, 47(3), 197–207.

Sternberg, R. J. (1997). *Thinking Styles*. Cambridge and New York: Cambridge University Press.

Stiglitz, J. E., Sen, A. and Fitoussi, J. (2009). Report by the Commission on the Measurement of Economic Performance and Social Progress, www.stiglitz-sen-fitoussi.fr.

Stinton, C., Elison, S. and Howlin, P. (2010). Mental health problems in adults with Williams syndrome. *American Journal on Intellectual and Developmental Disabilities*, 115, 3–18.

Stinton, C., Tomlinson, K. and Estes, Z. (2012). Examining reports of mental health in adults with Williams syndrome. *Research in Developmental Disabilities*, 33, 144–52.

Straetmans, J. M. J., van Schrojenstein Lantman-de Valk, H. M. J., Schellevis, F. G. and Dinant, G.-J. (2007). Health problems of people with intellectual disabilities: The impact for general practice. *British Journal of General Practice*, 57, 64–6.

Sturmey, P. (2007). Diagnosis of mental disorders in people with intellectual disabilities. In N. Bouras and G. Holt (eds.), *Psychiatric and Behavioural Disorders in Intellectual and Developmental Disabilities*. Cambridge University Press, pp. 3–23.

Sturmey, P. R., Lee, R. and Robek, A. (2003). *Substance-related Disorders in Persons with Mental Retardation*. New York: National Association for the Dually Diagnosed Press.

Sutherland, G., Couch, M. A. and Iacono, T. (2002). Health issues for adults with developmental disability. *Research in Developmental Disabilities*, 23, 422–45.

Swaine, J. G., Dababnah, S., Parish, S. L., Luken, K. (2013). Family caregivers' perspectives on barriers and facilitators of cervical and breast cancer screening for women with intellectual disability. *Intellectual and Developmental Disabilities,* 51(1), 12.

Symons, F. J., Shinde, S. K. and Gilles, E. (2008). Perspectives on pain and intellectual disability. *Journal of Intellectual Disability Research*, 52, 275–86.

Taggart, L., McLaughlin, D., Quinn, B. and Milligan, V. (2006). An exploration of substance abuse in people with intellectual disabilities. *Journal of Intellectual Disability Research*, 50, 588–97.

Tatochenko, V., Fedorov, A., Studenikin, V. and Zubovich, A. (2006). O chastote diagnostiki perinatalnovo porazheniya ZNS i svyasannih s nim lekarstvennih nagruskah [Frequency of diagnosis of perinatal brain injury and associated drug therapy] [In Russian]. *Meditsinskii Nauchnii i Uchebno-methodicheskii Zhurnal*, 30, 72–9, www.medic-21vek.ru/rubric/element.php?IBLOCK_ID=45andSECTION_ID=245andELEMENT_ID=2107; accessed 21 November 2010.

Taylor, J. L., Lindsay, W.R., Hastings, R.P., Hatton, C. (Ed.). (2013). *Psychological therapies for adults with intellectual disabilities*. Chichester: Wiley-Blackwell.

Taylor, J. L., Lindsay, W. R., Hastings, R. P. and Hatton, C.-P. (eds.). (2013). *Psychological Therapies for Adults with Intellectual Disabilities*. Chichester: Wiley.

Tellegen, C. L. and Sanders, M. R. (2013). Stepping Stones Triple-P Positive Parenting Program for children with disability: A systematic review and meta-analysis. *Research in Developmental Disabilities*, 34, 1556–71.

Temple, V. A., Foley, J. T. and Lloyd, M. (In press). Body mass index of adults with intellectual disability participating in Special Olympics by world region. *Journal of Intellectual Disabilities Research*.

The Information Centre for Health and Social Care. (2012). *Community Care Statistics 2010–11: Social Services Activity Report, England. Annexe A – National Tables*. Leeds: The Information Centre for Health and Social Care.

The Marmot Review. (2010). *Fair Society, Healthy Lives: Strategic Review of Health Inequalities in England Post-2010*. London: The Marmot Review.

Thillai, M. (2010). Respiratory diseases. In J. O'Hara, J. E. McCarthy and N. Bouras (eds.), *Intellectual Disability and Ill Health: A Review of the Evidence*. Cambridge University Press, pp. 78–87.

Thomas, C. (2007). *Sociologies of Disability and Illness. Contested Ideas in Disability Studies and Medical Sociology*. Basingstoke: Palgrave Macmillan.

Thomas, G. R. K. and Kerr, M.-P. (2011). Longitudinal follow-up of weight change in the context of a community-based health promotion programme for adults with an intellectual disability. *Journal of Applied Research in Intellectual Disabilities*, 24, 381–7.

Thomas, K., Bourke, J., Girdler, S. et al. (2011). Variation over time in medical conditions and health service utilisation of children with Down syndrome. *Journal of Pediatrics*, 158, 194–200.

Thomas, R. and Barnes, M. (2010). Life expectancy for people with disabilities. *Neurorehabilitation*, 27(2), 201–9.

Thomson, H., Atkinson, R., Petticrew, M. and Kearns, A. (2006). Do urban regeneration programmes improve public health and reduce health inequalities? A synthesis of the evidence from UK policy and practice. *Journal of Epidemiology and Community Health*, 60, 108–15.

Thomson, H., Thomas, S., Sellstrom, E. and Petticrew, M. (2013). Housing improvements for health and associated socio-economic outcomes. *Cochrane Database of Systematic Reviews* (2), CD008657.

Thornton, C. (1999). Effective healthcare for people with learning disabilities: A formal carers' perspective. *Journal of Psychiatric and Mental Health Nursing*, 6, 383–90.

Tiller, S., Wilson, K. I. and Gallagher, J. E. (2001). Oral health status and dental service use of adults with learning disabilities living in residential institutions and in the community. *Community Dental Health*, 18, 167–71.

Tilley, E.; Walmsley, J.; Earle, S.; Atkinson, D. (2012). 'The silence is roaring': sterilization, reproductive rights and women with intellectual disabilities. *Disability & Society, 27*(3), 14.

Torr, J. and Lee, L. (2010). Immune system diseases. In J. O'Hara, J. E. McCarthy and N. Bouras (eds.), *Intellectual Disability and Ill Health: A Review of the Evidence*. Cambridge University Press, pp. 47–60.

Totsika, V. and Hastings, R. P. (2012). How can population cohort studies contribute to our understanding of low-prevalence clinical disorders? The case of autism spectrum disorders. *Neuropsychiatry*, 2, 87–91.

Townsend, P. and Davidson, N. (1982). *Inequalities in Health: The Black Report*. Harmondsworth: Penguin.

Tracy, J. and Hosken, R. (1997). The importance of smoking education and preventative health strategies for people with intellectual disability. *Journal of Intellectual Disability Research*, 41, 6.

Trent, J. W. (1994). *Inventing the Feeble Mind: A History of Mental Retardation in the United States*. Berkeley, CA: University of Calfornia Press.

Truesdale-Kennedy, M., Taggart, L. and McIlfatrick, S. (2011). Breast cancer knowledge among women with intellectual disabilities and their experiences of receiving breast mammography. *Journal of Advanced Nursing*, 67, 1294–304.

Tsiouris, J. A. (2010). Pharmacotherapy for aggressive behaviours in persons with intellectual disabilities: Treatment or mistreatment? *Journal of Intellectual Disabilities Research*, 54, 1–16.

Tuffrey-Wijne, I., Bernal, J., Hubert, J., Butler, G. and Hollins, S. (2010). Exploring the lived experiences of people with learning disabilities who are dying of cancer. *Nursing Times*, 106, 15–18.

Tuffrey-Wijne, I., Hogg, J. and Curfs, L. (2007). End of life and palliative care for people with intellectual disabilities who have cancer or other life-limiting illness: A review of the literature and available resources. *Journal of Applied Research in Intellectual Disabilities*, 20, 331–44.

Turk, V., Kerry, S., Corney, R., Rowlands, G., Khattran, S. (2010). Why some adults with intellectual disability consult their general practitioner more than others. *Journal of Intellectual Disability Research*, 54, 10.

Turk, V., Kerry, S., Corney, R., Rowlands, G. and Khattran, S. (2010). Why some adults with intellectual disability consult their general practitioner more than others. *Journal of Intellectual Disability Research*, 54, 833–42.

Turk, V., Khattran, S., Kerry, S., Corney, R. and Painter, K. (2012). Reporting of health problems and pain by adults with an intellectual disability and by their carers. *Journal of Applied Research in Intellectual Disabilities*, 25, 155–65.

Turner, H. A., Finkelhor, D. and Ormrod, R. (2006). The effect of lifetime victimization on the mental health of children and adolescents. *Social Science and Medicine*, 62, 13–27.

Turner, S. and Robinson, C. (2010). *Health Checks for People with Learning Disabilities: Implications and Actions for Commissioners*. Durham: Improving Health and Lives: Learning Disabilities Observatory.

Tyler, C. V. J., Snyder, C. W. and Zyzanski, S. (2000). Screening for osteoporosis in community-dwelling adults with mental retardation. *Mental Retardation*, 38, 316–21.

Tymchuk, A. J., Lakin, K. C. and Luckasson, R. (2001). Life at the margins: Intellectual, demographic, economic, and social circumstances of adults with mild cognitive limitations. In A. J. Tymchuk, K. C. Lakin and R. Luckasson (eds.), *The Forgotten Generation: The Status and Challenges of Adults with Mild Cognitive Limitations*. Baltimore, MD: Brookes.

Tyrer, F. and McGrother, C. (2009). Cause-specific mortality and death certificate reporting in adults with moderate to profound intellectual disabilities. *Journal of Intellectual Disability Research*, 53, 898–904.

Uchino, B. N. (2006). Social support and health: A review of physiological processes potentially underlying links to disease outcomes. *Journal of Behavioral Medicine*, 29, 377–87.

Uchino, B. N., Cacioppo, J. T. and Kiecolt-Glaser, J. K. (1996). The relationship between social support and physiological processes: A review with emphasis on underlying mechanisms and implications for health. *Psychological Bulletin*, 119, 488–531.

Ungar, M. (2008). Resilience across cultures. *British Journal of Social Work*, 38, 218–35.

UNICEF. (2009). *Innocenti Social Monitor 2009. Child Well-Being at a Crossroads: Evolving Challenges in Central and Eastern Europe and the Commonwealth of Independent States*. Florence: UNICEF Innocenti Research Centre.

UNICEF. (2011). *The State of the World's Children 2011: Adolescence – An Age of Opportunity*. New York: UNICEF.

UNICEF. (2012). *The State of the World's Children: Children in an Urban World*. New York: UNICEF.

United Nations. (2003). *Standard Rules on the Equalization of Opportunities of Persons with Disabilities*. New York: United Nations.

United Nations. (2006). *Convention on the Rights of Persons with Disabilities*. New York: United Nations.

US Department of Health and Human Services. (2002a). *Closing the Gap: A National Blueprint to Improve the Health of Persons with Mental Retardation*. Rockville, MD: US Department of Health and Human Services.

US Department of Health and Human Services. (2002b). *Report of the Surgeon General's Conference on Health Disparities and Mental Retardation. Closing the Gap*. Rockville, MD: US Department of Health and Human Services.

Van de Poel, E., Hosseinpoor, A. R., Speybroeck, N., Van Ourtia, T. and Vega, J. (2008). Socio-economic inequality in malnutrition in developing countries. *Bulletin of the World Health Organization*, 86, 282–91.

van de Wouw, E., Evenhuis, H. M. and Echteld, M. A. (2012). Prevalence, associated factors and treatment of sleep problems in adults with intellectual disability: A systematic review. *Research in Developmental Disabilities*, 33, 1310–32.

Van Laecke, E. (2008). Elimination disorders in people with intellectual disability. *Journal of Intellectual Disabilities Research*, 52, 810.

van Schrojenstein Lantman-de Valk, H. (2005). Health in people with intellectual disabilities: Current knowledge and gaps in knowledge. *Journal of Applied Research in Intellectual Disabilities*, 18, 325–33.

van Schrojenstein Lantman-de Valk, H. M., Metsemakers, J. F., Haveman, M. J. and Crebolder, H. F. (2000). Health problems in people with intellectual disability in general practice: A comparative study. *Family Practice*, 17, 405–7.

van Schrojenstein Lantman-de Valk, H. and Walsh, P. (2008). Managing health problems in people with intellectual disabilities. *British Medical Journal*, 1408–12.

van Splunder, J., Stilma, J. S., Bernsen, R. M. D. and Evenhuis, H. M. (2004). Prevalence of ocular diagnoses found on screening 1539 adults with intellectual disabilities. *Ophthalmology*, 111, 1457–63.

van Splunder, J., Stilma, J. S., Bernsen, R. M. D. and Evenhuis, H. M. (2006). Prevalence of visual impairments in adults with intellectual disabilities in the Netherlands: Cross-sectional study. *Eye*, 20, 1004–10.

Wade, C, Llewellyn, G. and Matthews, J. (2011). Modeling contextual influences on parents with intellectual disability and their children. *American Journal on Intellectual and Developmental Disabilities*, 116, 419–37.

Wagemans, A. and Cluitmans, J. (2006). Falls and fractures: A major health risk for adults with intellectual disabilities in residential settings. *Journal of Policy and Practice in Intellectual Disabilities*, 3, 136–8.

Waldfogel, J., Craigie, T. and Brooks-Gunn, J. (2010). Fragile families and child well-being. *The Future of Children*, 20, 87–112.

Wang, M., Schalock, R. L., Verdugo, M. A. and Jenaro, C. (2010). Examining the factor structure and hierarchical nature of the quality of life construct. *American Journal on Intellectual and Developmental Disabilities*, 115(3), 218–33. DOI: 10.1352/1944-7558-115.3.218.

Ward, K. M., Windsor, R., Atkinson, J.P. (2012). A process evaluation of the Friendships and Dating Program for adults with developmental disabilities: Measuring the fidelity of program delivery. *Research in Developmental Disabilities, 33*, 7.

Warburg, M. (2001). Visual impairment in adult people with intellectual disability: Literature review. *Journal of Intellectual Disability Research*, 45, 424–38.

Waters, E., de Silva-Sanigorski, A., Hall, B.-J. et al. (2011). Interventions for preventing obesity in children. *Cochrane Database of Systematic Reviews*, published online 7 December.

Watson, N., Thomas, C. and Roulstone, A. (eds.). (2012). *Routledge Companion to Disability Studies*. London: Routledge.

Wee, L. E., Koh, G. C.-H., Auyong, L. S. et al. (In press). Screening for cardiovascular disease risk factors at baseline and post intervention among adults with intellectual disabilities in an urbanised Asian society. *Journal of Intellectual Disabilities Research*.

Wegman, H. L. and Stetler, C. (2009). A meta-analytic review of the effects of childhood abuse on medical outcomes in adulthood. *Psychosomatic Medicine*, 71, 805–12.

Welinder, L. G. and Baggesen, K. L. (2012). Visual abilities of students with severe developmental delay in special needs education – a vision screening project in Northern Jutland, Denmark. *Acta Ophthalmologica*, 90, 721–6.

Wells, J., Clark, K.D., Sarno, K. (2012). A computer-based interactive multimedia program to reduce HIV transmission for women with intellectual disability. *Journal of Intellectual Disability Research,* 56(4), 11.

Wells, M. B., Turner, S., Martin, D. M. and Roy, A. (1995). Health gain through screening – coronary heart disease and stroke: Developing primary healthcare services for people with intellectual disability. *Journal of Intellectual and Developmental Disability*, 22, 251–63.

Werner, E. and Smith, R. (1992). *Overcoming the Odds: High-Risk Children from Birth to Adulthood*. New York: Cornell University Press.

Westerinen, H., Kaski, M., Virta, L., Almqvist, F. and Iivanainen, M. (2007). Prevalence of intellectual disability: A comprehensive study based on national registers. *Journal of Intellectual Disability Research*, 51, 715–25.

Whitaker, S. (2004). Hidden learning disability. *British Journal of Learning Disabilities*, 32, 139–43.

White, M., Adams, J. and Heywood, P. (2009). How and why do interventions that increase health overall widen inequalities within populations? In S. J. Babones (ed.), *Social Inequality and Public Health*. Bristol: Policy Press, pp. 65–82.

Whitehead, M. (1992). The concepts and principles of equity and health. *International Journal of Health Services*, 22, 429–45.

Whitehead, S. J. and Ali, S. (2010). Health outcomes in economic evaluation: The QALY and utilities. *British Medical Bulletin*, 96, 5–21.

Whitfield, M., Langan, J. and Russell, O. (1996). Assessing general practitioners' care of adult patients with learning disability: case-control study. *Quality in Healthcare*, 5, 31–55.

WHO. (2010). *Better Health, Better Lives: Children and Young People with Intellectual Disabilities and Their Families. Transfer from Institutions to the Community. Bucharest, Romania, 17-26 November 2010*. Copenhagen: World Health Organization Regional Office for Europe.

Wilkenfeld, B. F. and Ballan, M.S. (2011). Educators' attitudes and beliefs towards the sexuality of individuals with developmental disabilities. *Sexuality and Disability*, 29, 11.

Wilkinson, K. M. and Hennig, S. (2007). The state of research and practice in augmentative and alternative communication for children with developmental/intellectual disabilities. *Mental Retardation and Developmental Disabilities Research Reviews*, 13, 58–69.

Wilkinson, R. G. (2005). *The Impact of Inequality*. New York: The New Press.

Wilkinson, R. G. and Pickett, K. E. (2009). *The Spirit Level: Why More-Equal Societies Almost Always Do Better*. London: Penguin.

Williams, S., Calnan, M. and Dolan, A. (2007). Explaining inequalities in health: Theoretical, conceptual and methodological agendas. In E. Dowler and N. Spencer (eds.), *Challenging Health Inequalities: From Acheson to 'Choosing Health'*. Bristol: The Policy Press.

Willis, D. S. et al. (2008). Breast cancer screening in women with learning disabilities: Current knowledge and considerations. *British Journal of Learning Disabilities*, 36, 171–84.

Willis, D. S., Wishart, J. G. and Muir, W. J. (2010). Carer knowledge and experiences with menopause in women with intellectual disabilities. *Journal of Policy and Practice in Intellectual Disabilities*, 7, 42–8.

Wilson, D. and Haire, A. (1990). Healthcare screening for people with mental handicap living in the community. *British Medical Journal*, 301, 1379–81.

Withers, P., Ensum, I., Howarth, D., Krall, P., Thomas, D., Weekes, D., Winter, C., Mulholland, A., Dindjer, T., Hall, J. (2001). A psychoeducational group for men who have sex with men. *Journal of Applied Research in Intellectual Disabilities*, 14(4), 14.

Wolfensberger, W. (1975). *The Origin and Nature of Our Institutional Models*. Syracuse: Human Policy Press.

Woodhouse, J. M. (2010). Eye diseases and visual impairment. In J. O'Hara, J. E. McCarthy and N. Bouras (eds.), *Intellectual Disability and Ill Health: A Review of the Evidence*. Cambridge University Press, pp. 146–55.

Woodhouse, M., Ryan, B., Davies, N. and McAvinchey, A. (2012). *A Clear Vision: Eye-care for Children and Young People in Special Schools in Wales*. Cardiff: Cardiff University.

Wolff, J. (2009). Cognitive disability in a society of equals. *Metaphilosophy*, 40(3–4), 402–415.

World Bank. (2011). *World Development Report 2011: Conflict, Security, and Development*. Washington, DC: World Bank.

Wolff, J. (2011). *Ethics and public policy : a philosophical inquiry*. Milton Park, Abingdon, Oxon, England ; New York: Routledge.

Wolff, J., & De-Shalit, A. (2007). *Disadvantage*. Oxford and New York: Oxford University Press.

World Health Organization. (1996). *ICD-10 Guide for Mental Retardation*. Geneva: World Health Organization.

World Health Organization. (2001). *International Classification of Functioning, Disability and Health*. Geneva: World Health Organization.

World Health Organization. (2004). *ICD-10: International Statistical Classification of Diseases and Related Health Problems (Tenth Revision; 2nd edn)*. Geneva: World Health Organization.

World Health Organization. (2007a). *Atlas: Global Resources for Persons with Intellectual Disabilities*. Geneva: World Health Organization.

World Health Organization. (2007b). *International Classification of Functioning, Disability and Health – Children and Youth Version. ICF-CY*. Geneva: World Health Organization.

World Health Organization. (2008). *Closing the Gap in a Generation: Health Equity through Action on the Social Determinants of Health. Final Report of the Commission on the Social Determinants of Health*. Geneva: World Health Organization.

World Health Organization. (2009). *Global Health Risks: Mortality and Burden of Disease Attributable to Selected Major Risks*.

World Health Organization. (2011a). *Rio Political Declaration on Social Determinants of Health* (www.who.int/sdhconference/declaration/en). Geneva: World Health Organization.

World Health Organization. (2011b). *World Report on Disability*. Geneva: World Health Organization.

World Health Organization. (2013). *The European Health Report 2012: Charting the Way to Well-being*. Copenhagen: WHO Regional Office for Europe.

World Health Organization and the World Bank. (2011). *World Report on Disability*. Geneva: World Health Organization.

World Health Organization Regional Office for Europe. (2010a). *European Declaration on the Health of Children and Young People with Intellectual Disabilities and their Families*. Copenhagen: World Health Organization Regional Office for Europe.

World Health Organization Regional Office for Europe. (2010b). *Interim First Report on Social Determinants of Health and the Health Divide in the WHO European Region*. Copenhagen: World Health Organization Regional Office for Europe.

Wright, D. and Digby, A. (1996). *From idiocy to mental deficiency : historical perspectives on people with learning disabilities*. London and New York: Routledge.

World Health Organization Regional Office for Europe. (2011). *Interim Second Report on Social Determinants of Health and the Health Divide in the WHO European Region.* Copenhagen: World Health Organization Regional Office for Europe.

Wright, D. and Digby, A. (1996). *From idiocy to mental deficiency : historical perspectives on people with learning disabilities.* London and New York: Routledge.

World Health Organization Regional Office for Europe. (2012). *Report on Social Determinants of Health and the Health Divide in the WHO European Region: Executive Summary.* Copenhagen: World Health Organization Regional Office for Europe.

Wu, C.-L. L., Lin, J.-D., Hu, J. et al. (2010). The effectiveness of healthy physical fitness programs on people with intellectual disabilities living in a disability institution: Six-month short-term effect. *Research in Developmental Disabilities*, 31, 713–17.

Yang, Q., Rasmussen, S. A. and Friedman, J. M. (2002). Mortality associated with Down's syndrome in the USA from 1983 to 1997: A population-based study. *Lancet*, 359, 1019–25.

Yeates, S. (1995). The incidence and importance of hearing loss in people with severe learning disability: The evolution of a service. *British Journal of Learning Disabilities*, 23, 79–84.

Yen, C.-F., Hsu, S.-W., Loh, C.-L., Fang, W.-H., Wu, C.-L., Chu, C.M., Lin, J.-D. (2012). Analysis of seasonal influenza vaccine uptake among children and adolescents with an intellectual disability. *Research in Developmental Disabilities*, 33, 7.

Zheng, X., Chen, R., Li, N. et al. (2012). Socio-economic status and children with intellectual disability in China. *Journal of Intellectual Disability Research*, 56, 212–20. DOI: 10.1111/j.1365-2788.2011.01470.x.

Index

accidents, 64
acquiescent responding, 47
adaptive behaviour, 18, 19
administrative records
  administrative prevalence, 41, 42–3
    'transition cliff', 42
  administrative sampling, 41
  coding accuracy, 46
  methods of recording, 46
    death certification, 46
    ICD-10 codes, 46
  research analysis of, 45–6
    bias of data, 46
    validity, 45–6
  see also 'hidden majority'
adolescents, 48, 92
adversity, exposure to
  biological embedding, 38
    allostatic load, 38
  environmental, *see* environmental factors
  mental health problems and, 72–3
  psychological pathways, 38
  resilience, 38
  social adversities, 70–5
  social pathways, 38
  socio-economic position, 37
aetiology (intellectual disability), 22–4
  biomedical approach, 22–3
  children
    early childhood, 23
    later childhood, 24
  environmental, *see* environmental factors
  multifactorial approach, 22–3
age 18 threshold, 18
age differences, prevalence rates, 21
alcohol misuse, 91
allostatic load, 38
ambulatory care-sensitive conditions, 77
anti-psychotic medication, 75–6, 96
  inappropriate use, 75–6

Australia, general health status, 53–8
autism, 46, 73–5

biomedical approach, aetiology/causes, 22–3
biopsychosocial model, 2–3, 4
  health inequalities conceptualisation, 3
bodily awareness, 81

cancer
  clinical interventions, 95
  healthcare services, 78
  in people with intellectual disabilities, 64
capabilities, 5
  combined, *see* combined capabilities
capability framework, 4–9
  central capabilities (importance), 8–9, 11
    comparison of models, 9
    spotlight indicators, 9
    UK policy, 9
  central focus, 4–6
  definitions, 5, 8
  health inequalities and, 5–8
  human rights, *see* human rights
  physical activity, 5–6
  pluralist, 5, 7
  quality-of-life approaches and, 6, 7
  self-definition, 5
  social justice, 5, 7
  well-being, 35
  see also substantial freedoms; well-being
capability security, 8
cardiovascular problems, 61
carers, as proxy responding, 47–9
causes of intellectual disability, *see* aetiology
central domains of life, 8–9, 11
challenging behaviours, 59, 74
  anti-psychotic drugs, inappropriate use, 75–6
children
  causes of intellectual disability, *see* aetiology
    (intellectual disability)

children (*cont.*)
  cognitive testing, 44
  disability prevalence, 31
  health measurement, 26
  health promotion, 89–90
  health status, 54
    with/without intellectual disability, 53
  inequalities (health), socially patterned, 24
  knowledge base development, 110–11
  long-lasting protective interventions, 99–100
  mental health and challenging behaviour, 58
  physical activity, capability framework, 5–6
  poor health, 52
  social gradients in prevalence, 23–4
  surveys, 44
classification (of intellectual disability), 18–19
  AAIDD, 18
  adaptive behaviour, 18, 19
  age 18 threshold, 18
  'hidden majority', *see* 'hidden majority'
  high-income countries, 18
  ICF, 2–3
  IQ, 18–19, 20
  mild, *see* 'hidden majority'
  models, 1–3
    capability framework, *see* capability
      framework
    mapping to health/health inequalities, 3–4
    see also biopsychosocial model; medical
      model; social model
coding accuracy, 46
cognitive testing, children, 44
combined capabilities, 5
  measurement of, 6
communication disorders, 61
community (social) networks, 78–9
consent, *see* informed consent
constipation, 62
constitutional factors, 80–1
corrosive disadvantage, 8
counselling, *see* health impact pyramid
  framework

death certification, 46
dementia, 59, 80
diet, *see* nutrition/diet
disability, 2, 32
  functioning and, 32–33
  human rights and, 32
  ICF, 28, 32
  impairment, health and, distinction
    between, 3

indicator of health, as an (inverse), 33
  measures of, 32
  prevalence, *see* prevalence
disability adjusted life years (DALYs), 33
discrimination, 67–8
  definitions, 69
  human rights and, 68
  knowledge base development, 112
  policy and legislation, 69–70
Down's syndrome
  health risks, 62–3, 80
  mortality and life expectancy, 49
  surgical interventions, 96
dysphagia, 62

education, *see* health impact pyramid
  framework
endocrine problems, 62–3
environmental factors, 2, 23
  environmental adversities, 36, 70–5
  indirect effects, 37
  life course approach, 37, 110–11
  living and working conditions, 70–8, 101–2
  material hazards, 36
  psychosocial hazards, 36
  regional and international variation, 20
  risk of exposure, 36–7
  see also socio-economic factors
epidemiology (intellectual disability), 19–24
  incidence, *see* incidence
  IQ as threshold, 20
  prevalence, *see* prevalence
  sampling and study design, 21
epilepsy, 59–60
exercise, *see* physical activity
exposure to adversity, *see* adversity, exposure to

falls, 64
fertile functioning, 8

gastro-oesophageal reflux disease (GORD), 62
gender differences, prevalence rates, 21
genitourinary and reproductive functions, 63
GPs
  financial incentives, 46, 98
  mental health problems, 58–9
gross domestic product (GDP), 4

haematological problems, 61
health, 25–39
  checks, 98–9
  conceptualisation and measurement, 25–35

children, 26
disability adjusted life years (DALYs), 33
general health status, 26–7
measurement methods, 25, 43–9
mortality and life expectancy, 26
prevalence of diseases/conditions, 27–9
quality adjusted life years (QALYs), 33
well-being, *see* well-being
definitions, 4, 25, 32
determinants of, 36–9
 exposure to adversity, *see* adversity,
  exposure to
 social, *see* social determinants of health
disability as indicator, 33
functioning and disability, 32–33
general health status, 26–7, 52–8
general indicators, 49–53
health functioning, 6
 minimum thresholds, 7
ICD and ICF classification systems, 27, 28
impact pyramid, *see* health impact pyramid
 framework
impairment/disability and, distinction
 between, 3
inequalities, *see* inequalities (health)
literacy, 81, 111–12
measurement, 25, 43–9
promotion, *see* health promotion
public health interventions, *see* public health
 interventions
screening, *see* health screening
surveys, *see* surveys (health)
health (of people with intellectual disabilities),
 40, 56, 80–1, 108–9
ambulatory care-sensitive conditions, 77
cancer, 64
cardiovascular conditions, 61, 80
children, *see* children
consent, health interventions, 85
constipation, 62
default decisions, 100–3
dysphagia, 62
endocrine conditions, 62–3
evidence-base, *see* research methodology
gastro-oesophageal reflux disease (GORD), 62
general health status, 52–8
general indicators, 49–53
genitourinary and reproductive functions, 63
haematological system, 61
health checks, 98–9
health impact pyramid, *see* health impact
 pyramid framework

health literacy and, 111–12
health promotion, *see* health promotion
health risk profile, 87
health screening, 76, 97, 99
 programmes, 97
inequality perspective, *see* inequalities
 (health)
mental functions, 58–60, 80
 see also mental health problems
mortality rates, *see* mortality and life
 expectancy
neuromusculoskeletal/movement-related
 functions, 63–4
 injuries, accidents and falls, 64
 osteoporosis, 63
 physical impairments, 63
obesity and, 81
oral health, 61–2
public health interventions, *see* public health
 interventions
respiratory disease, 61
secondary analysis, 43
sensory functions and pain, 60
skin conditions, 64
sleep disorders, 60, 81
specific health conditions and
 impairments, 53–65
vaccination, 97
voice and speech functions, 61
health impact pyramid framework, 84–5, 105–7,
 109–10
health risk profile, 87
'hidden majority', 85
level 1: counselling and education, 87–94
 diet, physical activity and weight
  reduction, 87–90
 mental health, *see* mental health problems
 oral health, 91–2
 sexual health, *see* sexual health
 smoking, alcohol and drug misuse, 90–1
level 2: clinical interventions, 94–6
 surgical interventions, 96
level 3: long-lasting protective interventions,
 96–100
level 4: healthy default decisions, 100–3
 public health, *see* public health
  interventions
level 5: socio-economic factors, *see* socio-
 economic factors
rainbow model comparison, 84
strengths, 85
health inequalities, *see* inequalities (health)

health promotion, 76
  children, 89–90
  factors influencing efficacy, 88–9
  interventions, 87–90
health screening, 76, 97, 99
  programmes, 97
healthcare services, 75–8
  barriers to, 75
  to clinical interventions, 94
  cancer, 78
  health promotion, *see* health promotion
  health screening, *see* health screening
  institutional settings, 74, 75–6
  primary care, *see* primary healthcare
  secondary healthcare, 77–8, 95
'hidden majority', 42–3, 64, 116
  health impact pyramid, 85
  knowledge base development, 111
  mild intellectual disability, 49
high-income countries, 18, 115–16
human rights
  capability framework, 8
  disability and, 32, 68–9
  discrimination and, 68
  social model approach, 2
hypothalamic disorders, 80
hypothalamic–pituitary–adrenal (HPA) axis, 38
hypothyroidism, 62–3

IAPT (Improving Access to Psychological
    Therapies), 93
identification (of people with intellectual
    disability), 44–5, 46
ill health, people with, *see* health (of people with
    intellectual disabilities)
impairment, 2
  disability, health, distinction between, 3
Improving Access to Psychological Therapies
    (IAPT), 93
incidence, 19, 20
income group, prevalence rates, 21
incontinence, 81
individual lifestyle factors, *see* lifestyle factors
individual model, *see* medical model
inequalities (health), 25–39, 66–82, 108
  addressing/reducing, 83–107
    health impact pyramid, *see* health impact
        pyramid framework
    public health, *see* public health perspective
  biopsychosocial model approach, 3
  capability framework and, *see* capability
      framework
  conceptualisations, 3

definition, 35
determinants, 36–9, 67–82
  constitutional factors, 80–1
  environmental conditions, 67–70
  healthcare services, *see* healthcare services
  lifestyle factors, *see* lifestyle factors
  living/working conditions,
      see environmental factors
  social and community networks, 78–9
  socio-economic/cultural, *see* socio-
      economic factors
frameworks, 66
  rainbow model, *see* rainbow model (of
      health)
measurement, 6
public health perspective, *see* public health
    perspective
socially patterned, 24
socio-economic inequalities and, 104
infant mortality rates, 26, 27, 28
informed consent
  health interventions, 85
  research methodology, 45
injuries, accidents and falls, 64
institutional settings, 74, 75–6
intellectual disability, 1–24
  bodily awareness, 81
  classification, *see* classification (of intellectual
      disability)
  definition/meanings, 18–19
  epidemiology, *see* epidemiology (intellectual
      disability)
  health issues in, *see* health (of people with
      intellectual disabilities)
  health literacy and, 111–12
  health screening, 97
  'hidden majority', *see* 'hidden majority'
  identification, 44–5, 46
  internal capabilities and, 19
  prevalence, *see* prevalence
  reasonable adjustments, *see* reasonable
      accommodations/adjustments
  records, *see* administrative records
  rights of people with, 114
  social construct, as a, 19
  'visible minority', 42–3
intelligence quotient (IQ), 18–19, 20
internal capabilities, intellectual disability and, 19
International Classification of Functioning,
    Disability and Health (ICF) (WHO),
    2–3, 28
  aim, 32
  definition of disability, 32

policy and practice, 4
International Statistical Classification of
      Diseases and Related Health Problems
      (ICD) (WHO), 27, 46

knowledge base development, 110–13

language disorders, 61
life course approach, 37, 110–11
life expectancy, *see* mortality and life expectancy
lifestyle factors, 79–80
literacy, health, 81, 111–12
living and working conditions, 70–8, 101–2
low- and middle-income countries, 20, 115

material hazards, 36
medical model, 1–2, 32
      health inequalities concept, 3
Mencap, definitions, discrimination, 69
mental health problems, 58–9, 80, 92–3
      anti-psychotic drugs, 75–6, 96
      dementia, 59, 80
      exposure to adverse life events, 72–3
      GP identification, 58–9
      health inequality reduction, 92–3
      identification of, 49, 58–9
      psychological interventions, 93
      social determinants, 59
      see also challenging behaviours
middle-income countries, 20, 115
mild intellectual disability, 49
      see also 'hidden majority'
minority ethnic status, 18–19, 22, 71
models, *see* classification (of intellectual
      disability)
mortality and life expectancy, 26, 29, 49–51
      cause of deaths, 51
      Down's syndrome, 49
      infant mortality rates, 26, 27, 28
      mild intellectual disability, 49
      moderate to severe intellectual disability, 49
      preventable or premature deaths, 50–1
      standardised, 50

Netherlands, general health status, 53–8
New Deal for Communities Programme, 100
nutrition/diet, 79
      interventions (reducing health inequalities),
            87–90, 101

obesity, 79, 81
      health inequalities and, 79
      prevalence, 30

weight reduction, inequality reduction, 81
older adults, primary healthcare, 77
oppression (societal), 2
oral health, 61–2, 91–2
osteoporosis, 63

pain, 60
physical activity, 79
      capability framework, 5–6
      health impact pyramid and, 87–90
      interventions, 89, 102–3
      public health interventions, 102–3
physical impairments, 63
pluralist
      capability framework, 5, 7
policy and practice
      changing, 113–15
            creating alliances, 114–15
            knowledge base, 114
            social model approach, 2
      discrimination, 69–70
      future, 110–15
      ICF, 4
      rights of intellectually disabled people, 114
      well-being indicators, 34–5
      see also knowledge base development
prevalence
      autism, 46
      disability, 32
            children, 31
            UK, 31
      intellectual disability, 19, 20–2
            administrative prevalence,
                  see administrative records
            competent/incompetent people, 20
            identification, 44–5, 46
            minority ethnic communities, 22
            socio-economic factors, 22
            variations in, 21–2
      knowledge base development, 112–13
      obesity, 30
      specific diseases/conditions, 27–9
prevention strategies, 83–4
primary healthcare, 77, 95
      older adults, 77
      unmet health needs, identification, 77
proxy responding, 47–9
psychological approach
      IAPT, 93
      to mental health problems, 93
      to well-being, 34
psychosocial hazards, 36
public health interventions, 100–1

public health interventions (*cont.*)
for general population, 102–3
outcomes, assessing, 86
physical activity, 102–3
smoking bans, 102
tobacco taxation, 102
public health perspective, 83–7
health impact pyramid, *see* health impact
pyramid framework
prevention strategies, 83–4
reasonable adjustments, 86

quality adjusted life years (QALYs), 33
quality-of-life framework, 6, 7, 11

rainbow model (of health), 66, 67, 109
comparison with health impact pyramid, 84
reasonable accommodations/adjustments, 113
clinical interventions, 95
health check provision, 77
public health context, 86
in research methodology, 47, 48
sampling, 45
research methodology, 40–9
consent, informed, 45
data collection, 43–9
acquiescent responding, 47
adolescents, 48
proxy responding, 47–9
records, *see* administrative records
response bias, 47
self-report, 47–9, 52
surveys (health), *see* surveys (health)
general health status, 52–8
health measurement, 43–9
health promotion interventions, 87
'hidden majority', 111
intervention outcomes, 86
sampling of participants, 41–3, 113
see also sampling of research participants
secondary analysis, 43
socio-economic position, 72
see also health impact pyramid framework
resilience, 38
respiratory disease, 61
response bias, 47

sampling of research participants, 41–3, 113
administrative samples, *see* administrative
records
intellectual disability identification, 44–5, 46

reasonable accommodations, *see* reasonable
accommodations/adjustments
skewed sample, 45
surveys, *see* surveys (health)
triangulation of data, 44–5
secondary analysis, 43
secondary healthcare, 77–8, 95
self-definition, capabilities approach, 5
self-efficacy, 38
self-report, 47–9, 52
sensory functions, 60
severe intellectual disability, mortality and life
expectancy, 49
sexual health, 80, 92
adolescents, 92
sexual violence, 92
short stature, 62
skin and related structures, 64
sleep disorders, 60, 81
smoking
bans, 102
cessation programmes, 90–1
tobacco taxation, 102
social and community networks, 78–9
social determinants of health, 38–9, 73–5, 112
mental health problems, 59
social mobility, 39
UK, 70
social justice, capabilities approach, 5, 7
social mobility, 39
social model, 2, 32
health/impairment/disability, distinction
between, 3
health inequalities conceptualisation, 3
socio-economic factors, 23–4, 67–70, 103–4
discrimination, *see* discrimination
health promotion, factors influencing, 88–9
interventions, 104
minority ethnic status and, 18–19, 22, 71
prevalence rate, 22
social adversities, 70–5
socio-economic inequalities, and health, 104
socio-economic position (SEP), 73
autism and, 73–5
implications, 71–3
methodological considerations, 72
risk of exposure to environmental
adversities, 37
speech functions, 61
spotlight indicators, 9, 17
Stepping Stones Triple-P intervention, 99–100

substance use, 80, 91
  health inequality reduction, 90–1
substantial freedoms, 5
  capability model, 5, 8
  measurement of, 6
  physical activity, 6
surveys (health), 43–5
  adults, 44–5
  children, 44
  large-scale, 43–5
  methodological challenges, 44
  sampling
    general population, 45
    intellectual disabilities, participants
        with, 44–5
  secondary analysis, 43

tobacco taxation, 102
'transition cliff', 42
Triple-P behavioural family intervention, 99–100

UK
  administrative records, 46
  children, health status, 53, 58
  disability prevalence, 31, 46
  general health status, 53–8
  GPs' financial incentives, 46
  legislation, 86
  mortality and life expectancy, 49, 51
  policy, central capabilities, 9

reasonable adjustments, 86
  social determinants of poor health, 70
  well-being indicators, 34–5
UN Convention on the Rights of Persons with
        Disabilities (UNCRPD), 11, 32, 69
underweight, 79
unmet health needs, identification of, 77
urban vs rural population, prevalence rates, 21
USA, incidence rates of intellectual
        disability, 20

vaccination, 97
validity, well-being measurement, 34
valuable capabilities, central domains of life, 11
'visible minority', 42–3, 113, 116
voice and speech functions, 61

weight reduction, 87–90
well-being, 33–5
  measurement, 33–4
    sensitivity and validity, 34–5
  social policy, implications for, 34–5
WHO
  definition of health, 32
  disability as a human rights issue, 68–9
  ICD, 27, 46
  quality-of-life framework, 11
women, genitourinary/reproductive
        functions, 63
working conditions, 70–8, 101–2